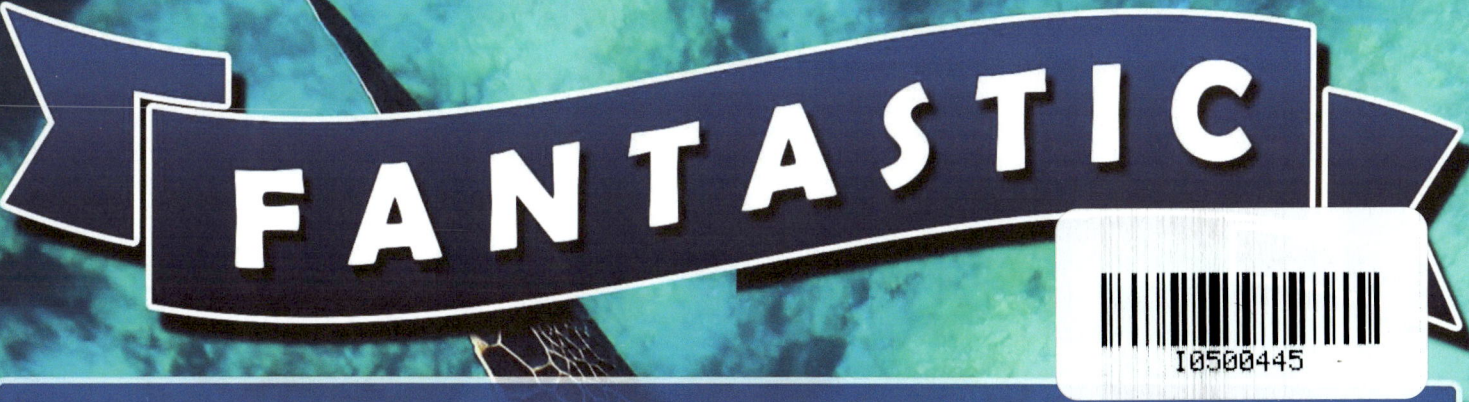

FANTASTIC

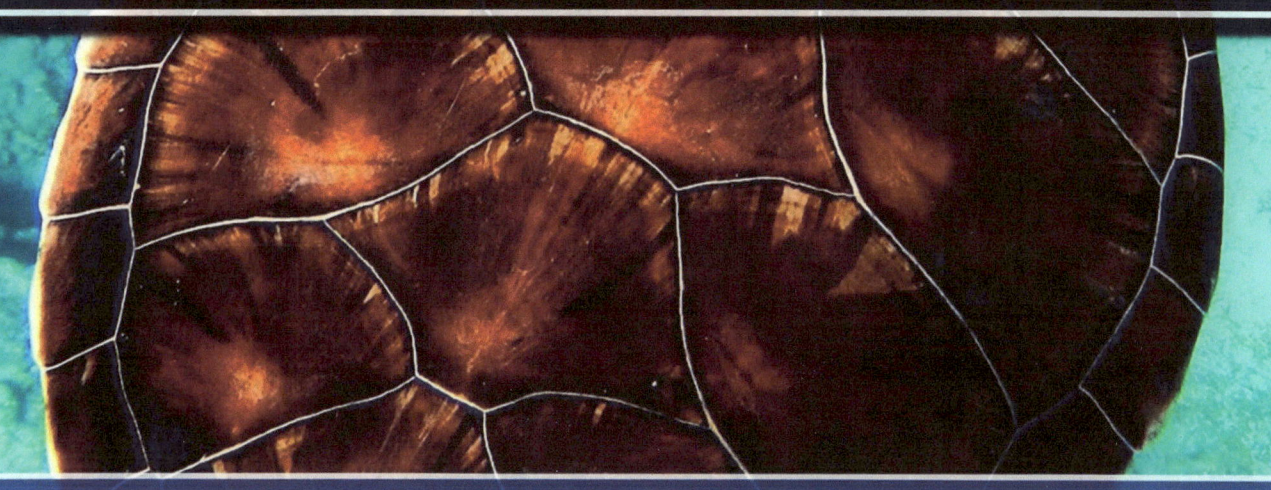

ANIMALS

40 FULL COLOR IMAGES

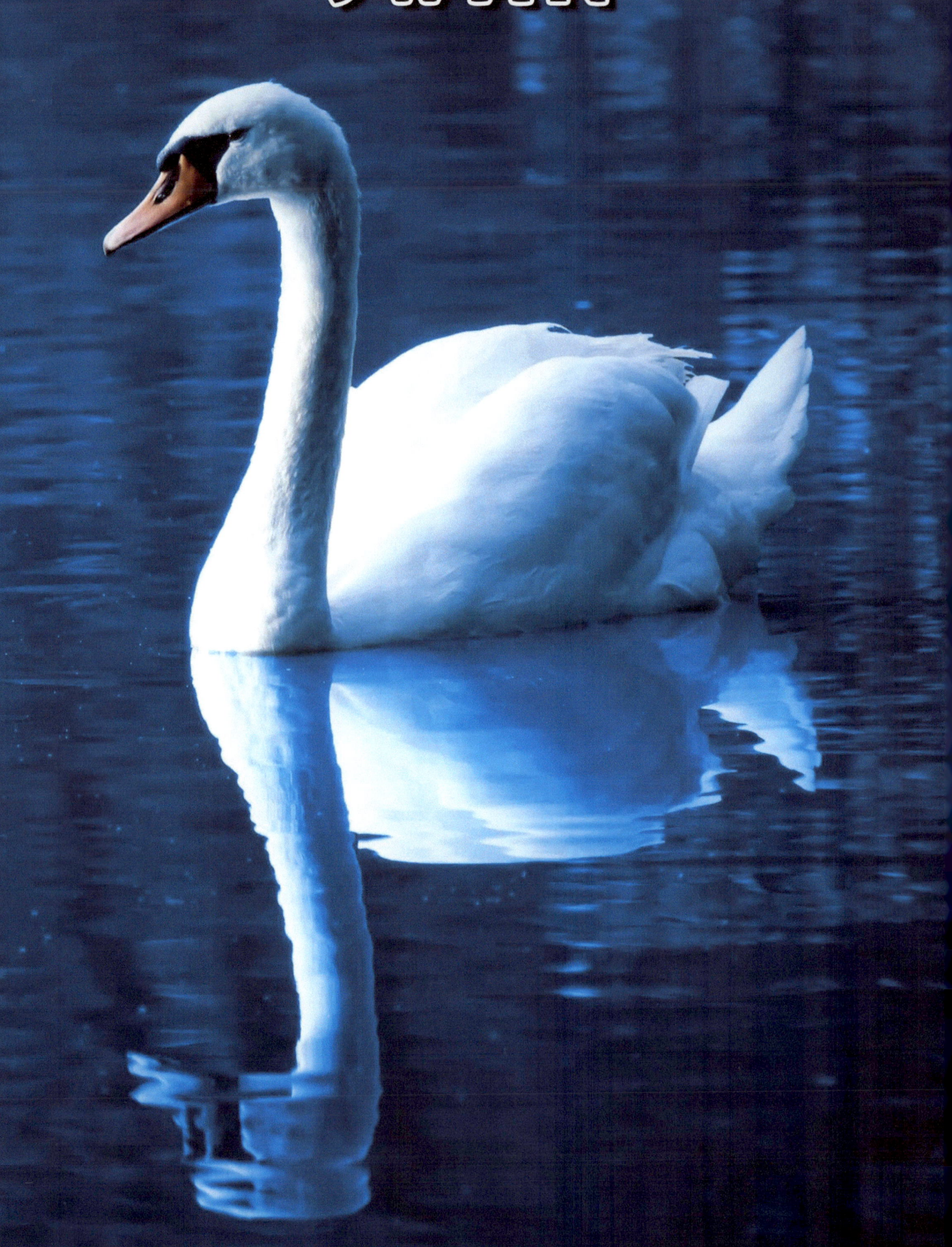

SWAN

ZEBRA

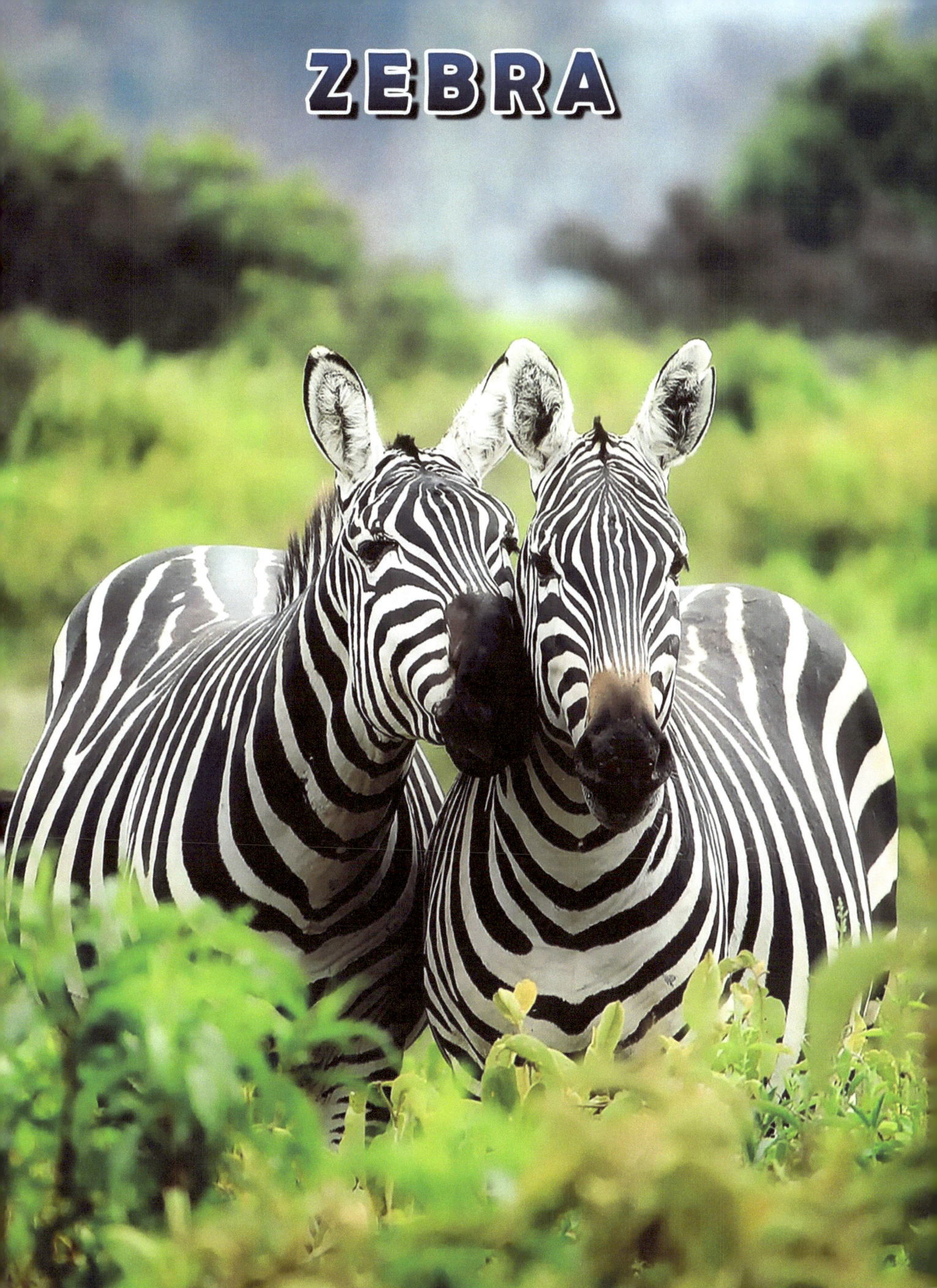

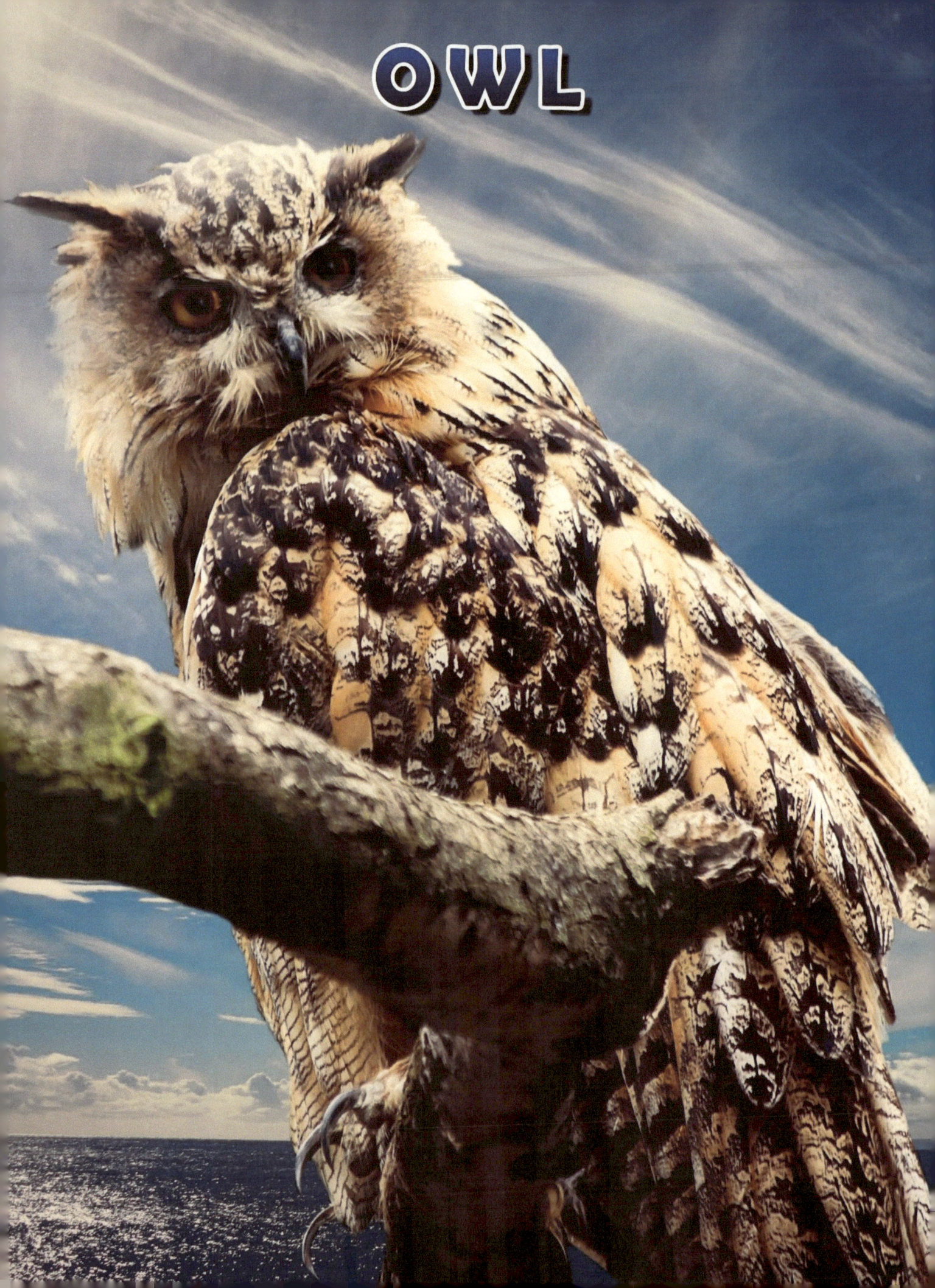

OWL

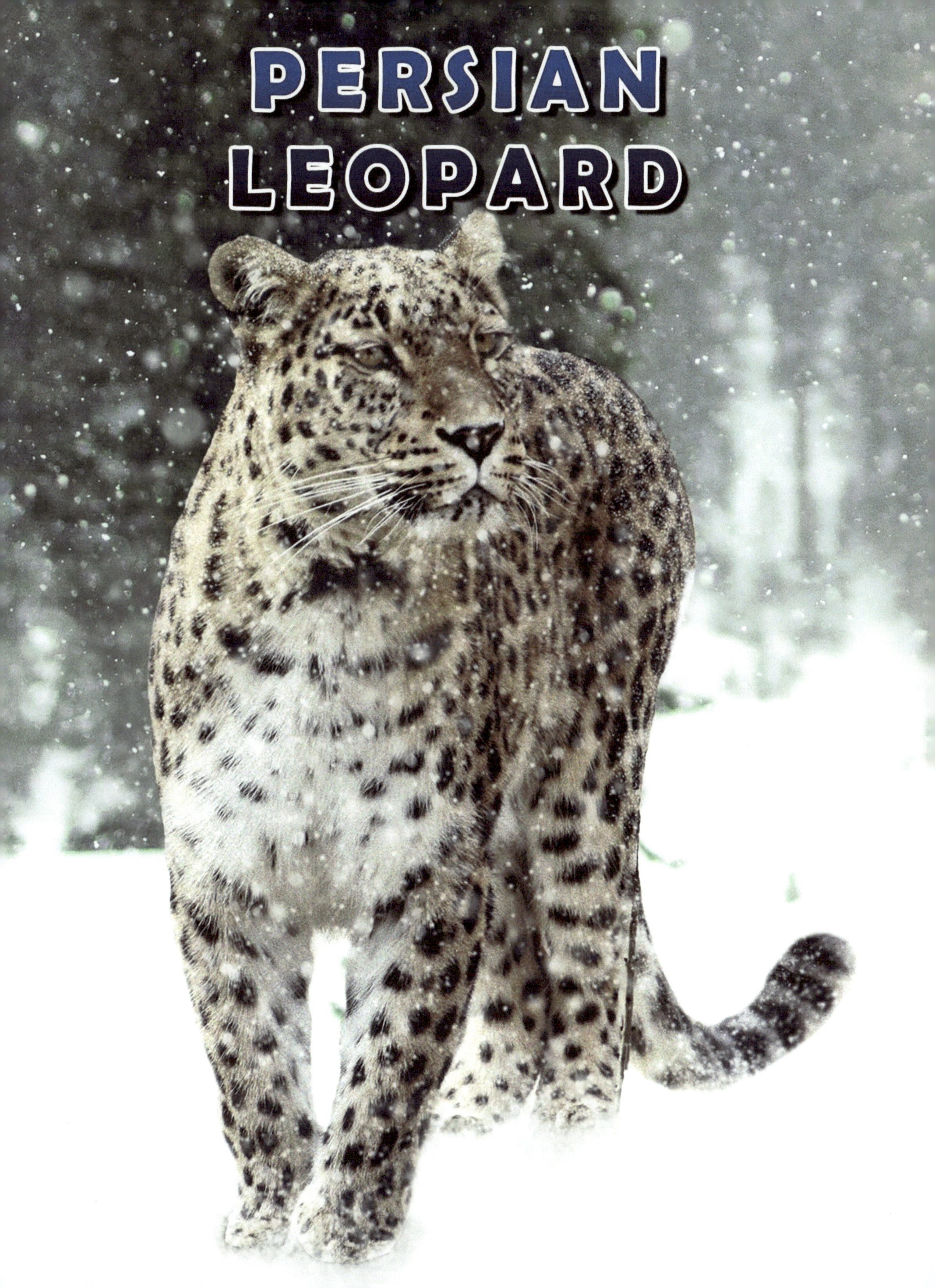

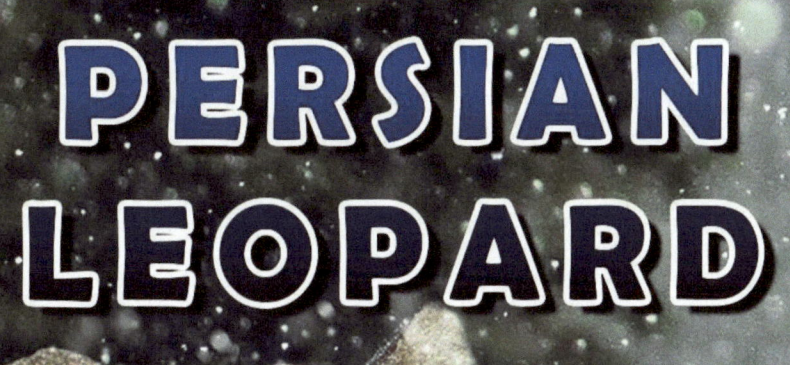

LEMUR

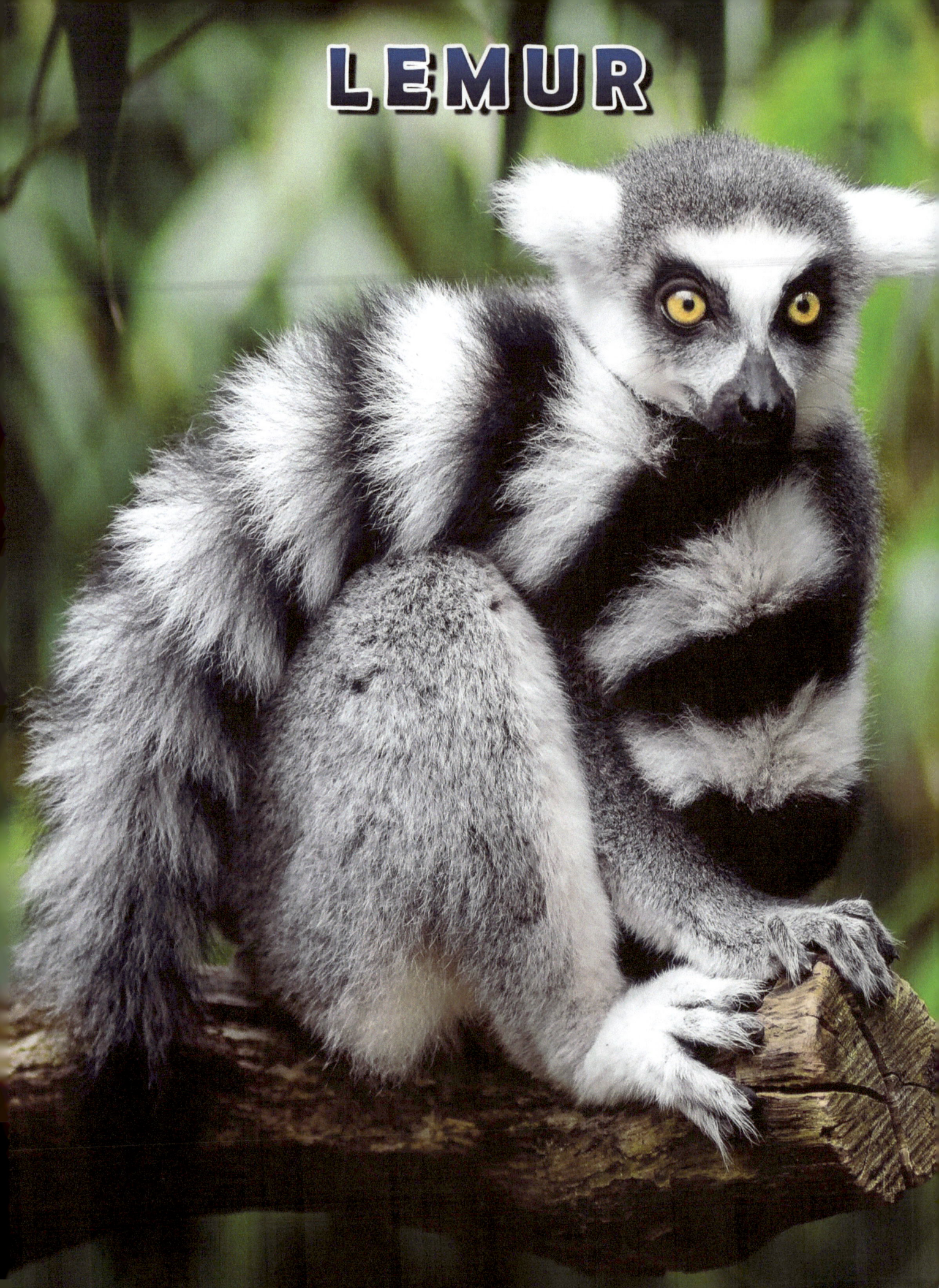

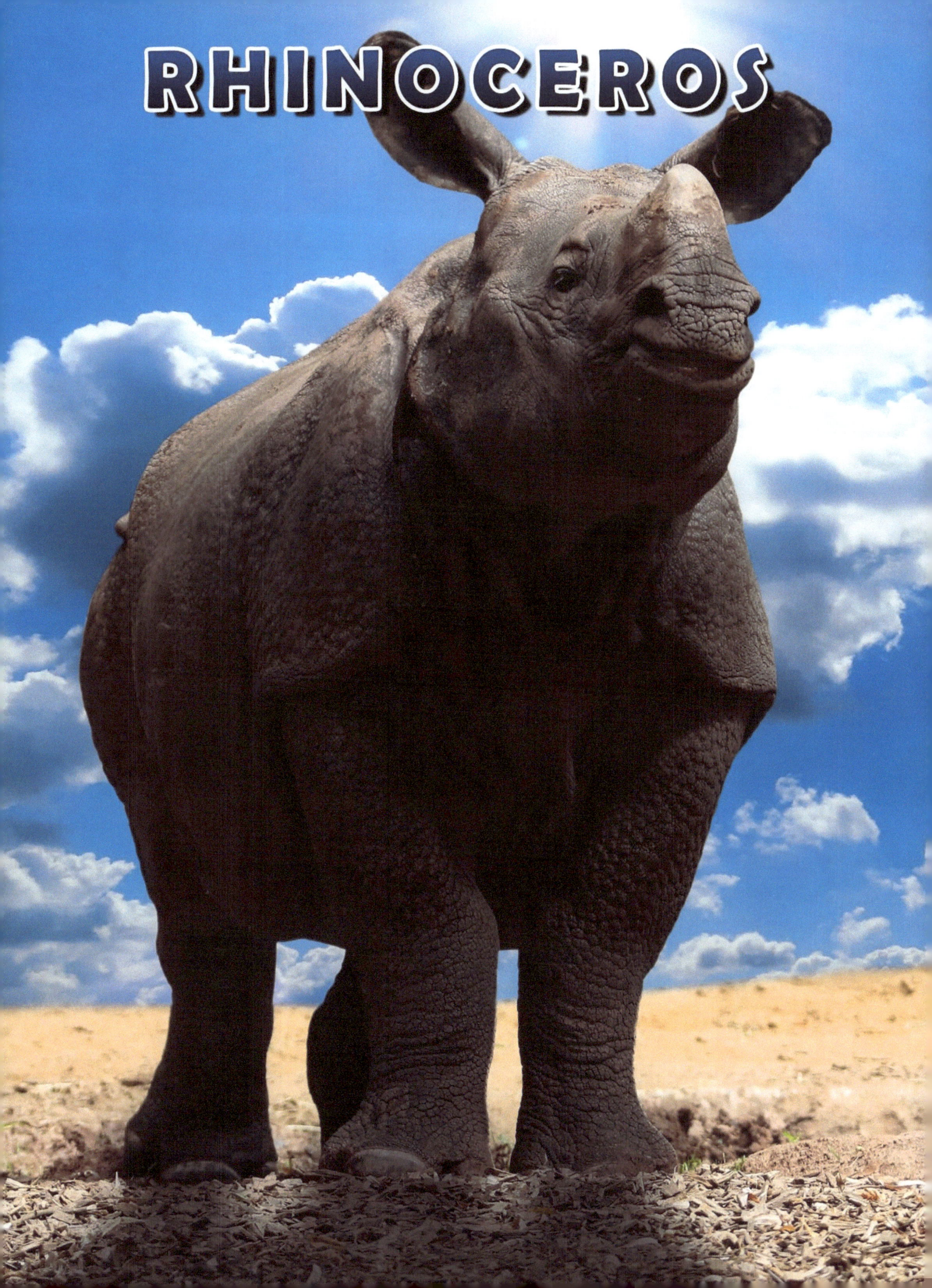

RHINOCEROS

CHIPMUNK

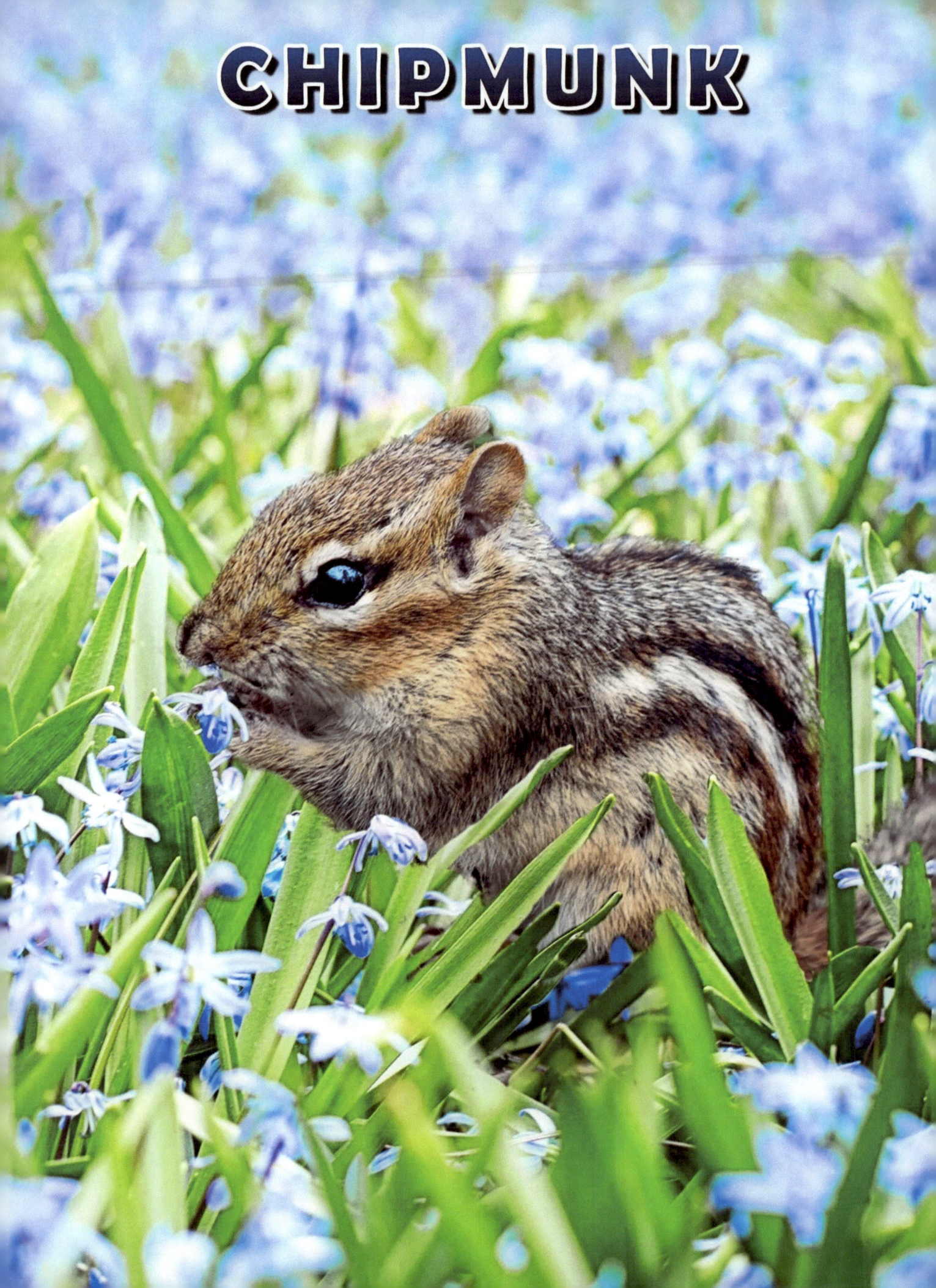

CHEETAH

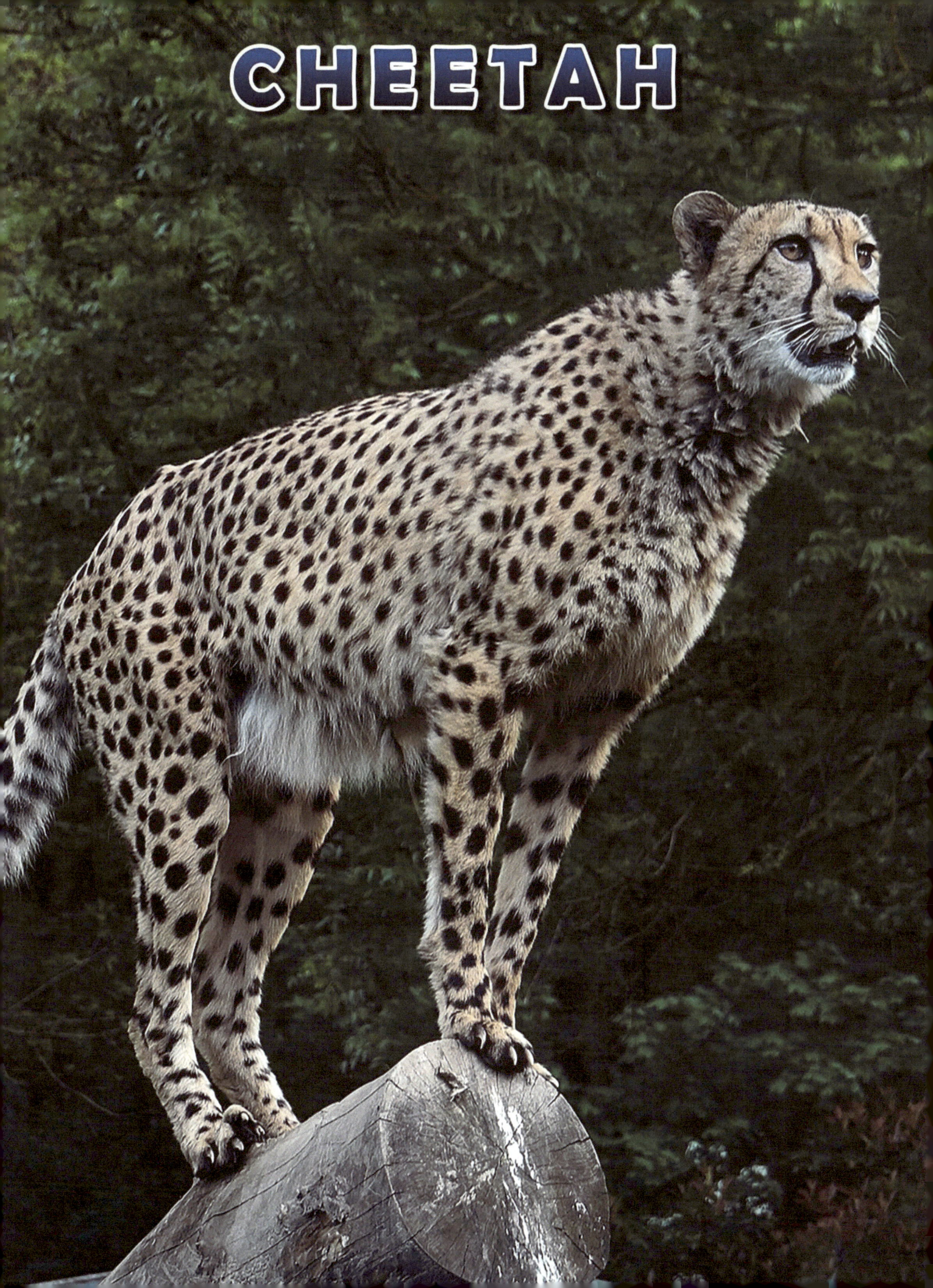

HEDGEHOG

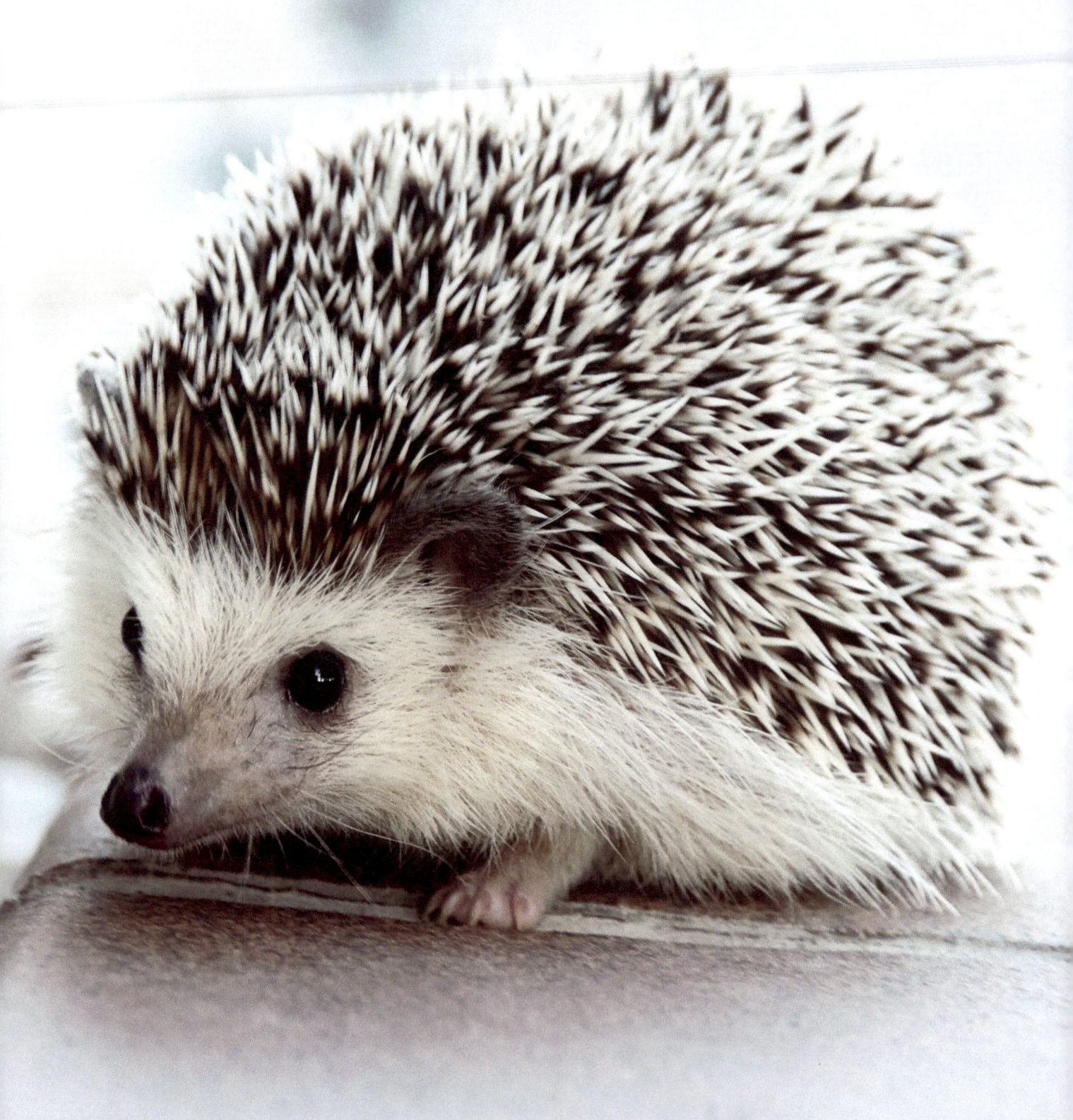

GIRAFFE

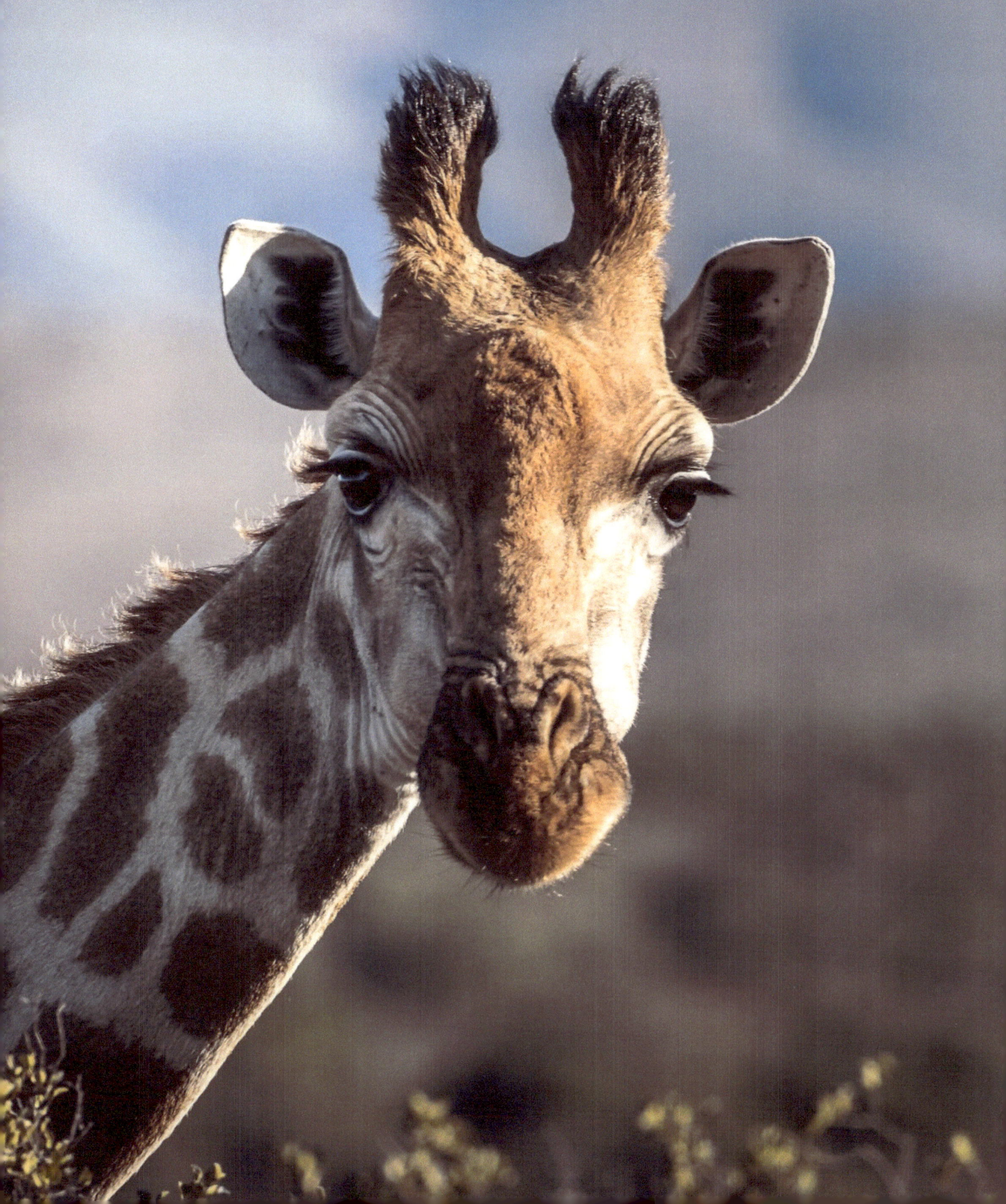

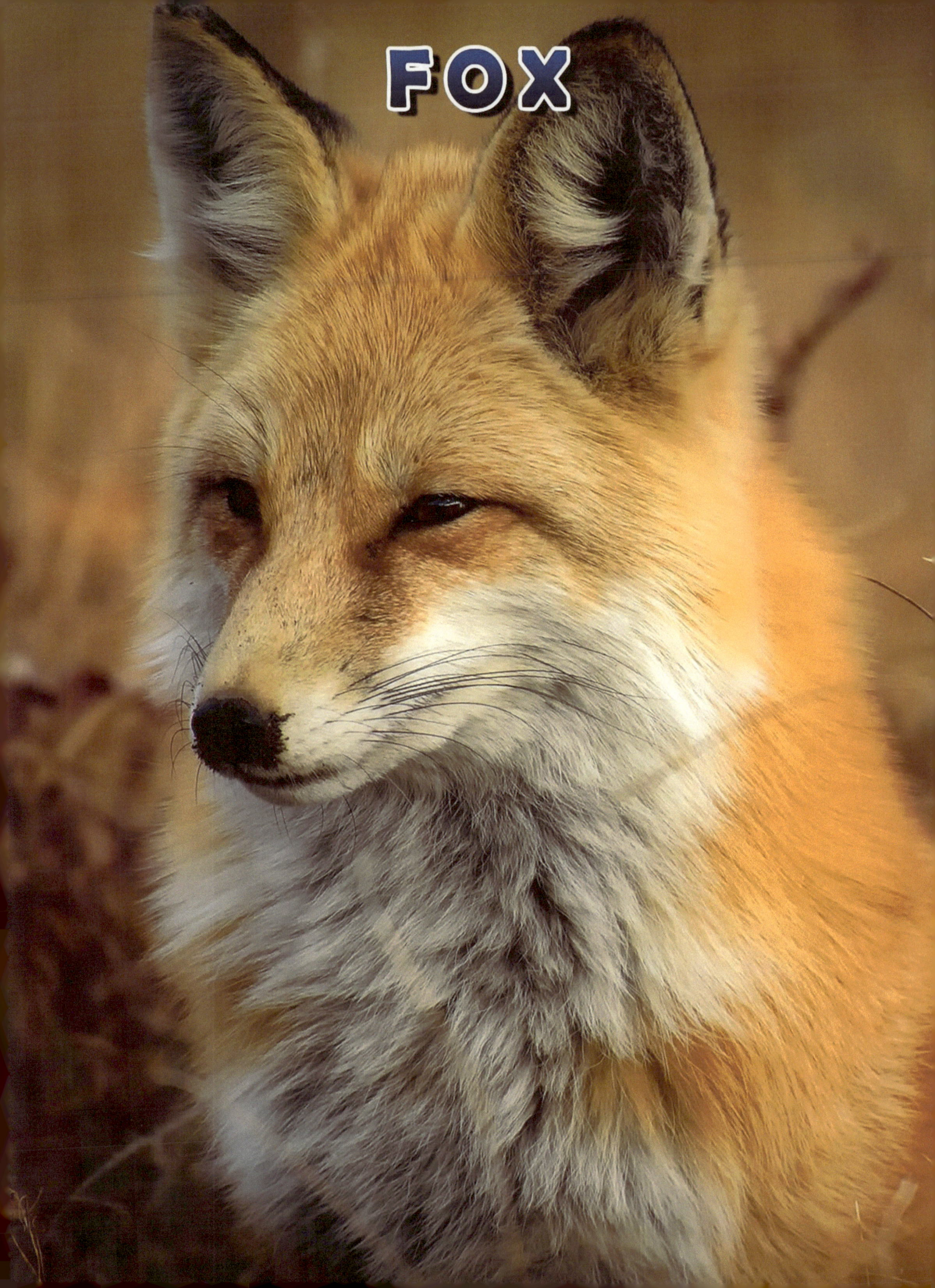

FOX

EMPEROR PENGUINS

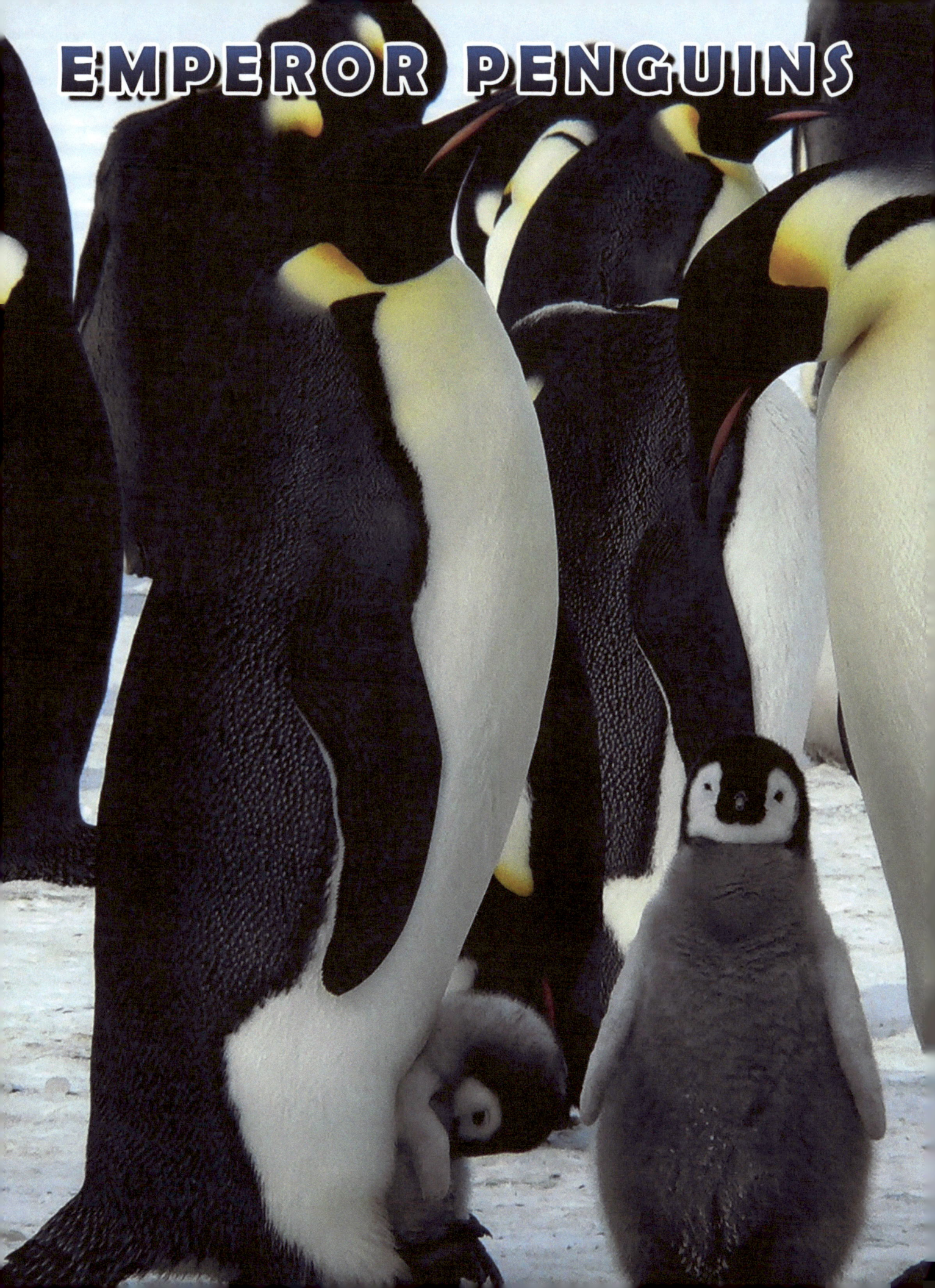

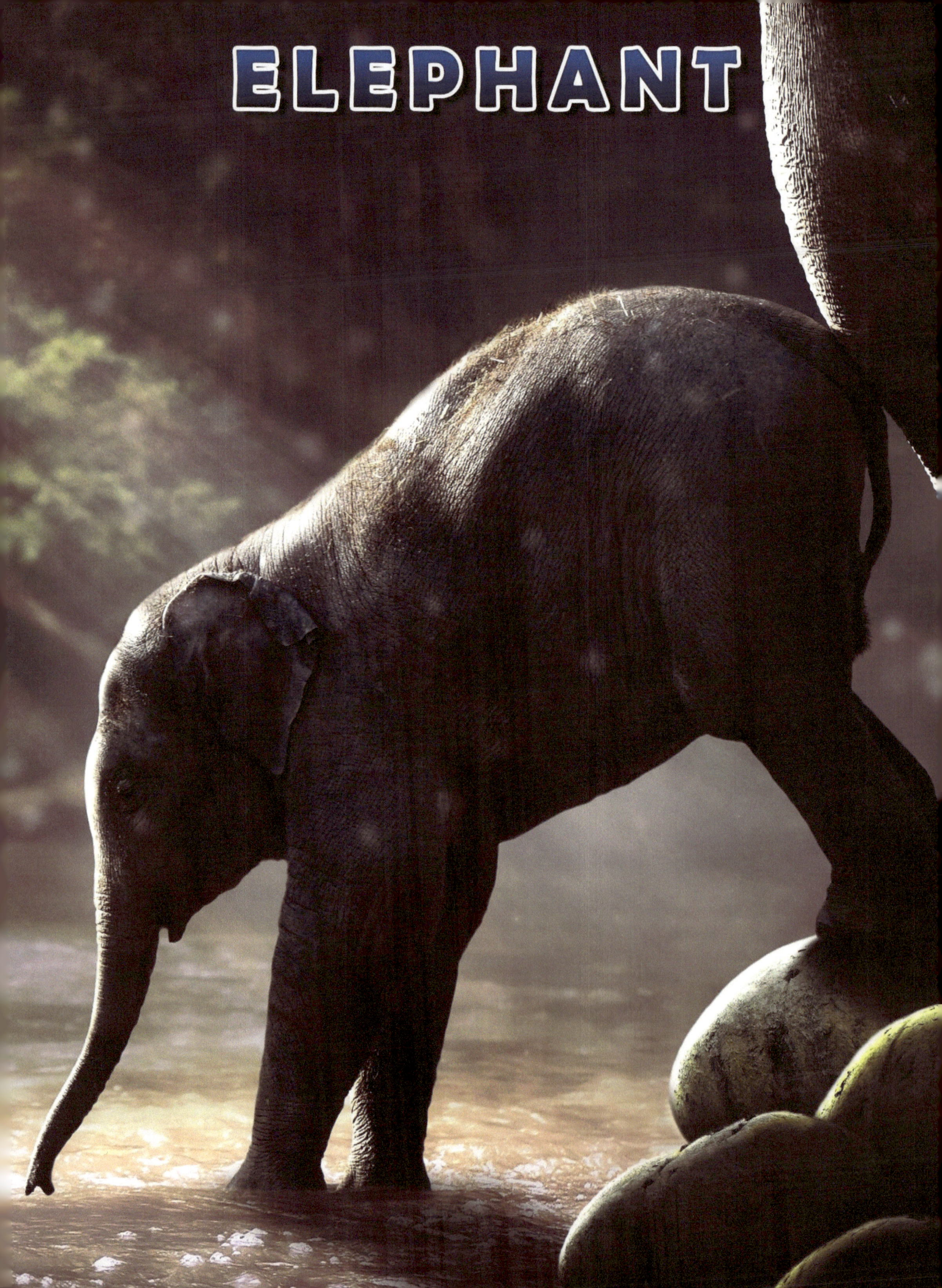

ELEPHANT

DOVE

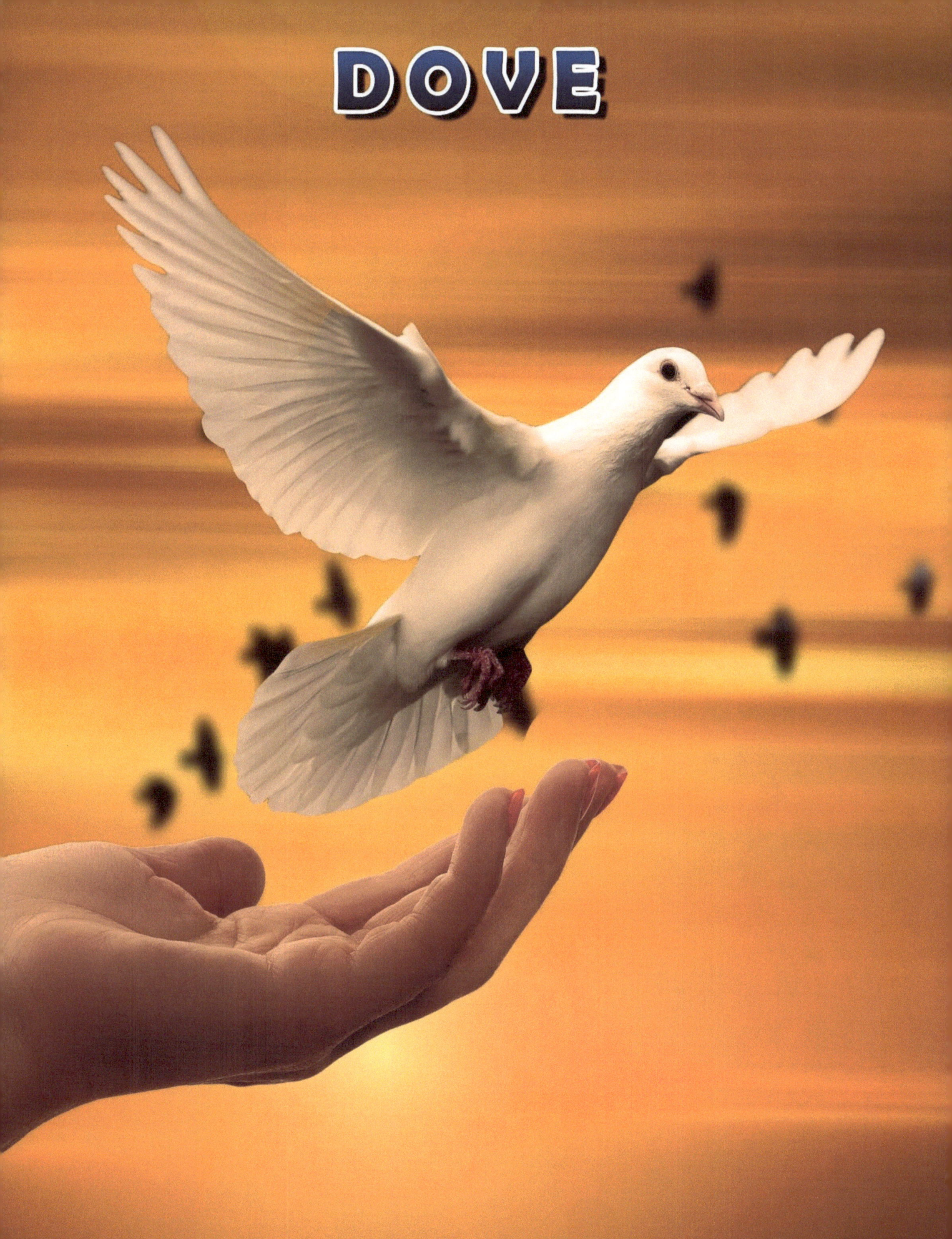

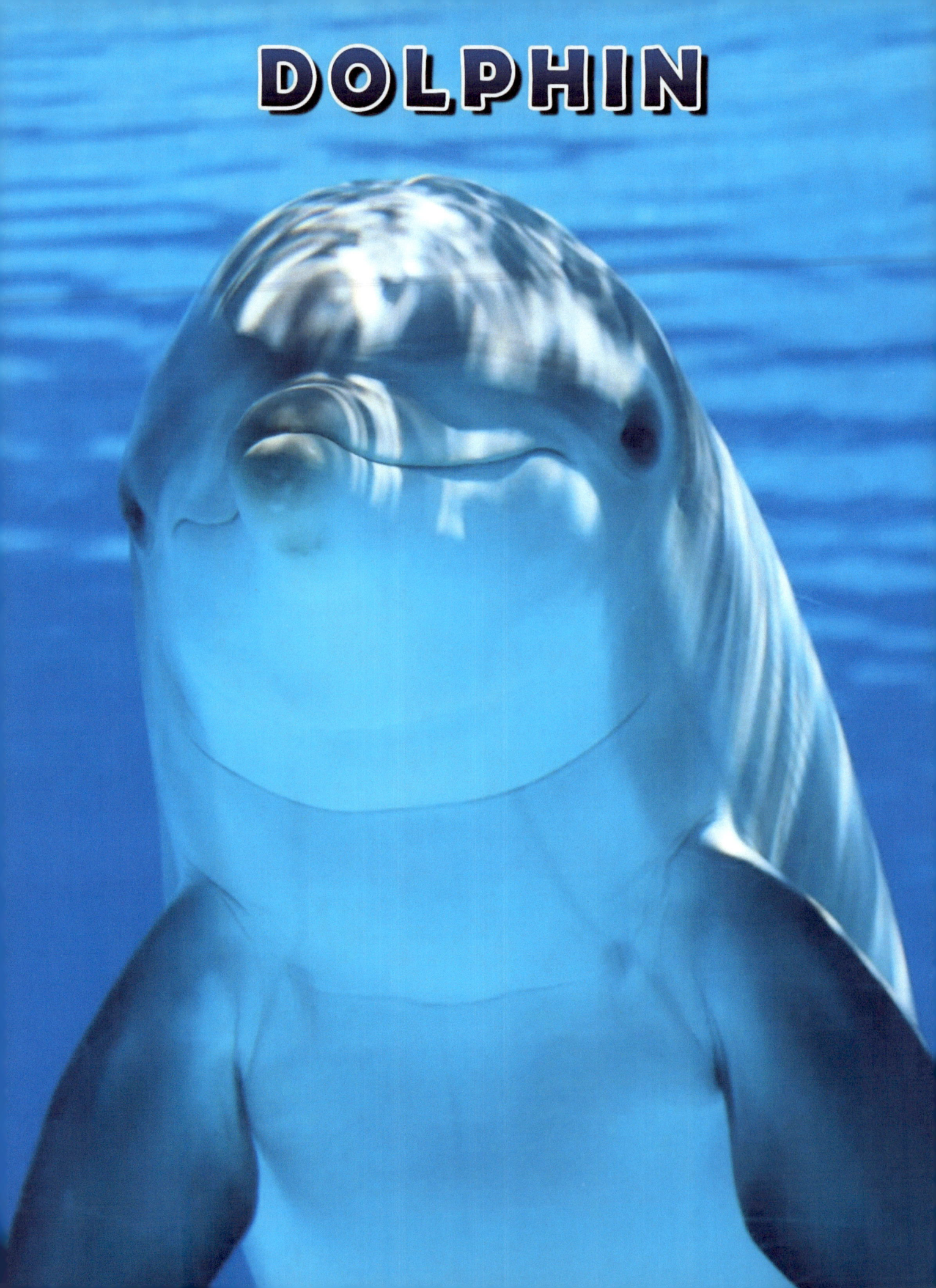

DOLPHIN

DOG

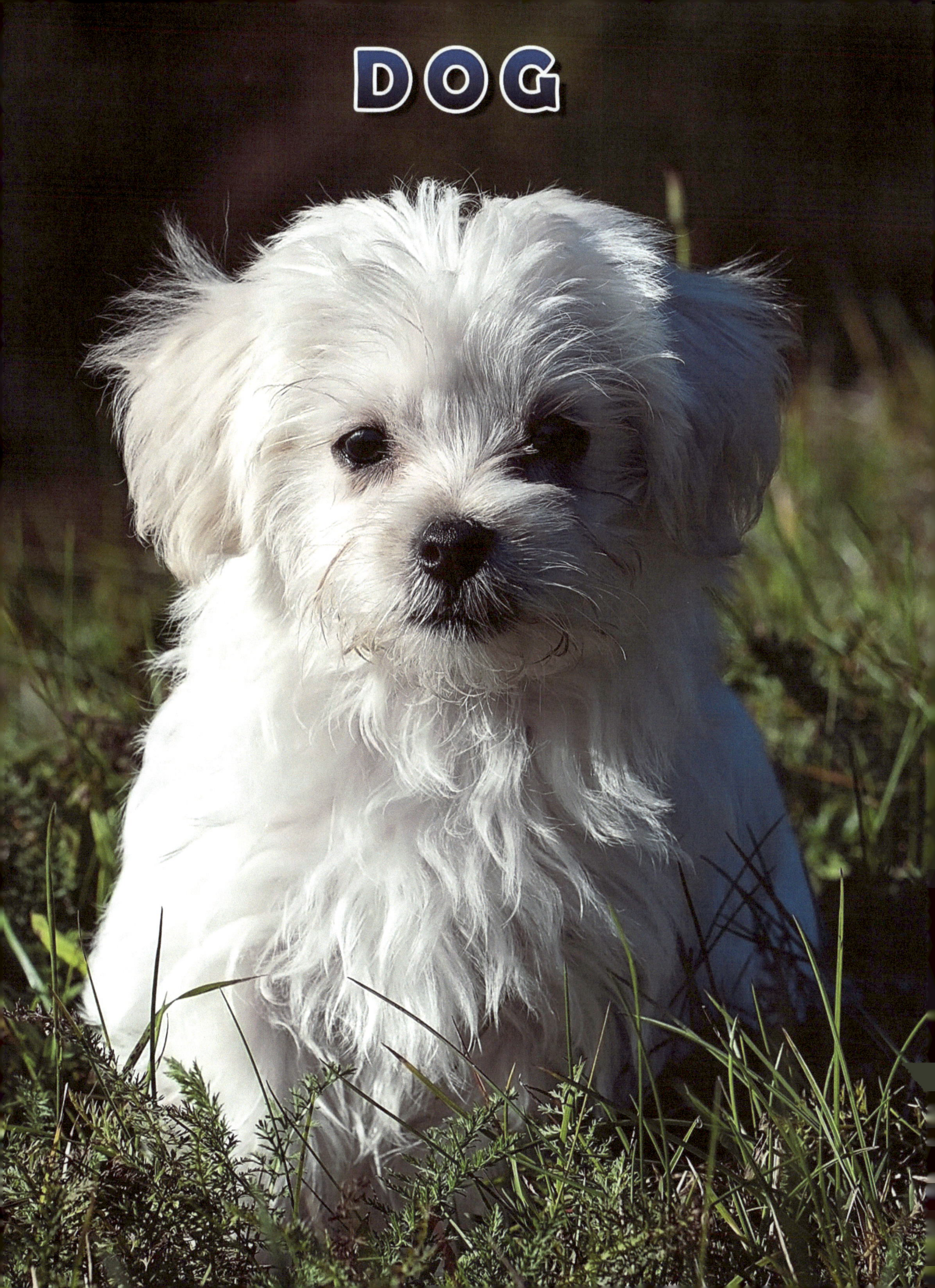

RED POMPADOUR COTINGA

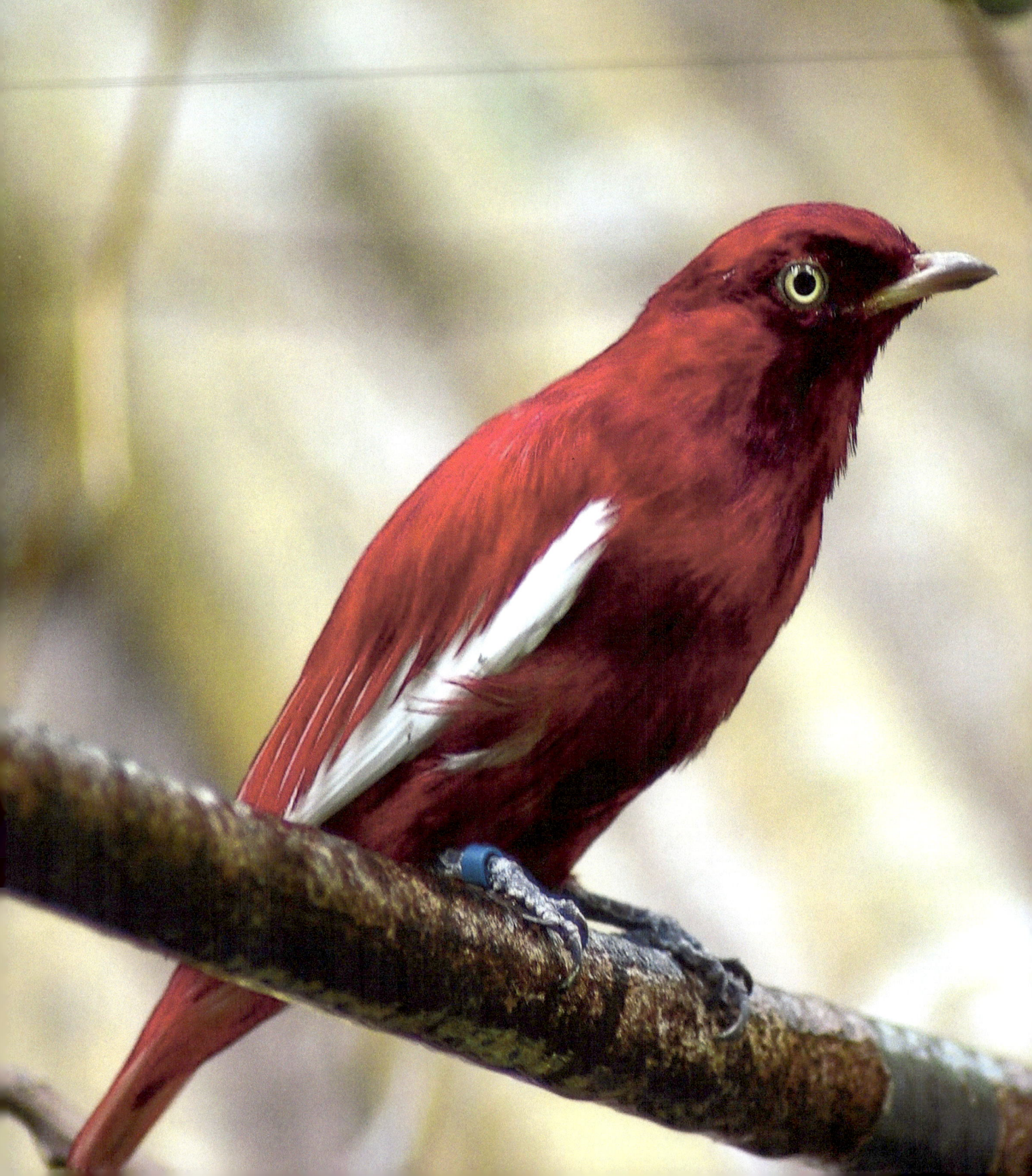

OCTOPUS

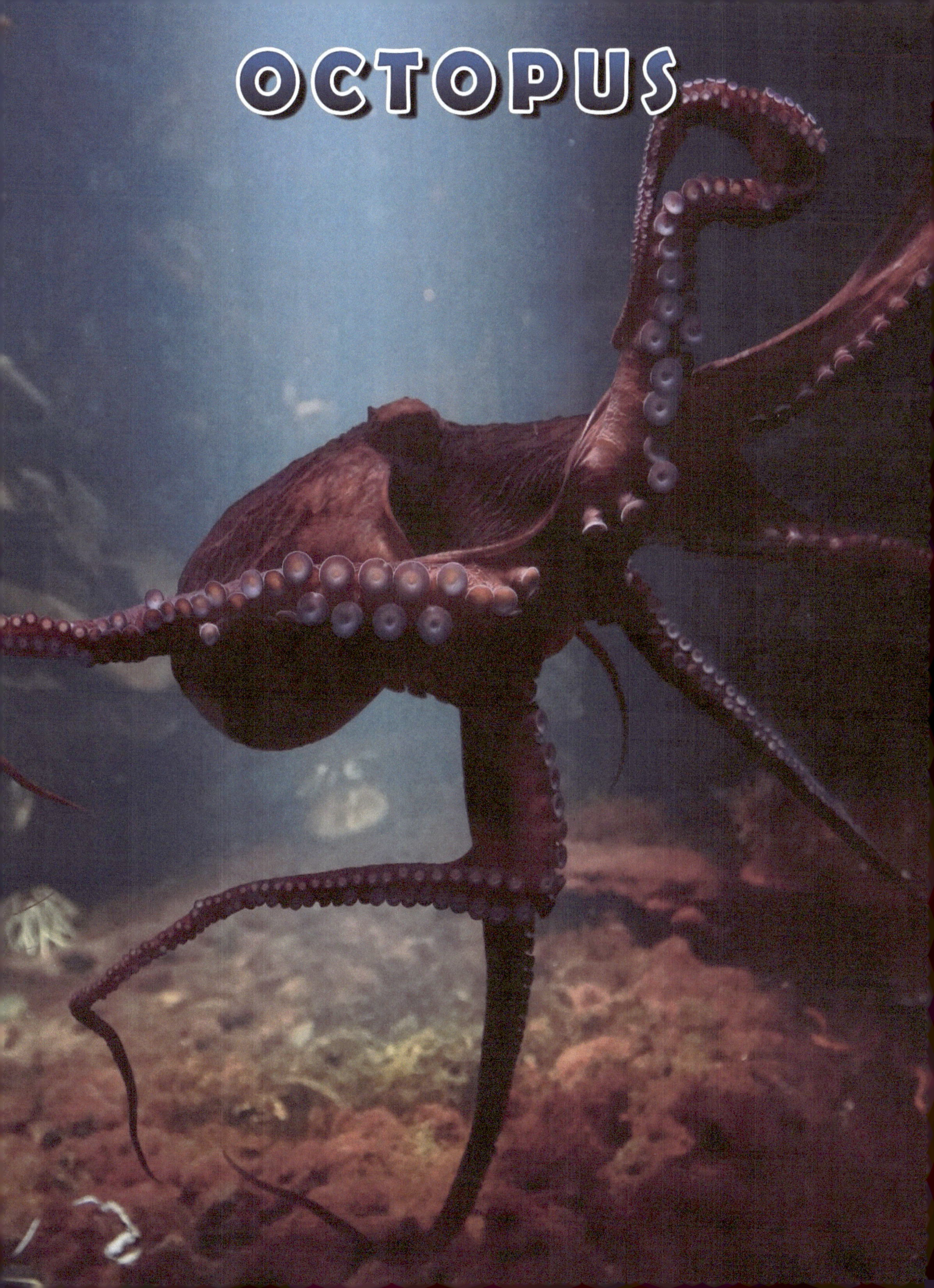

MANDRILL

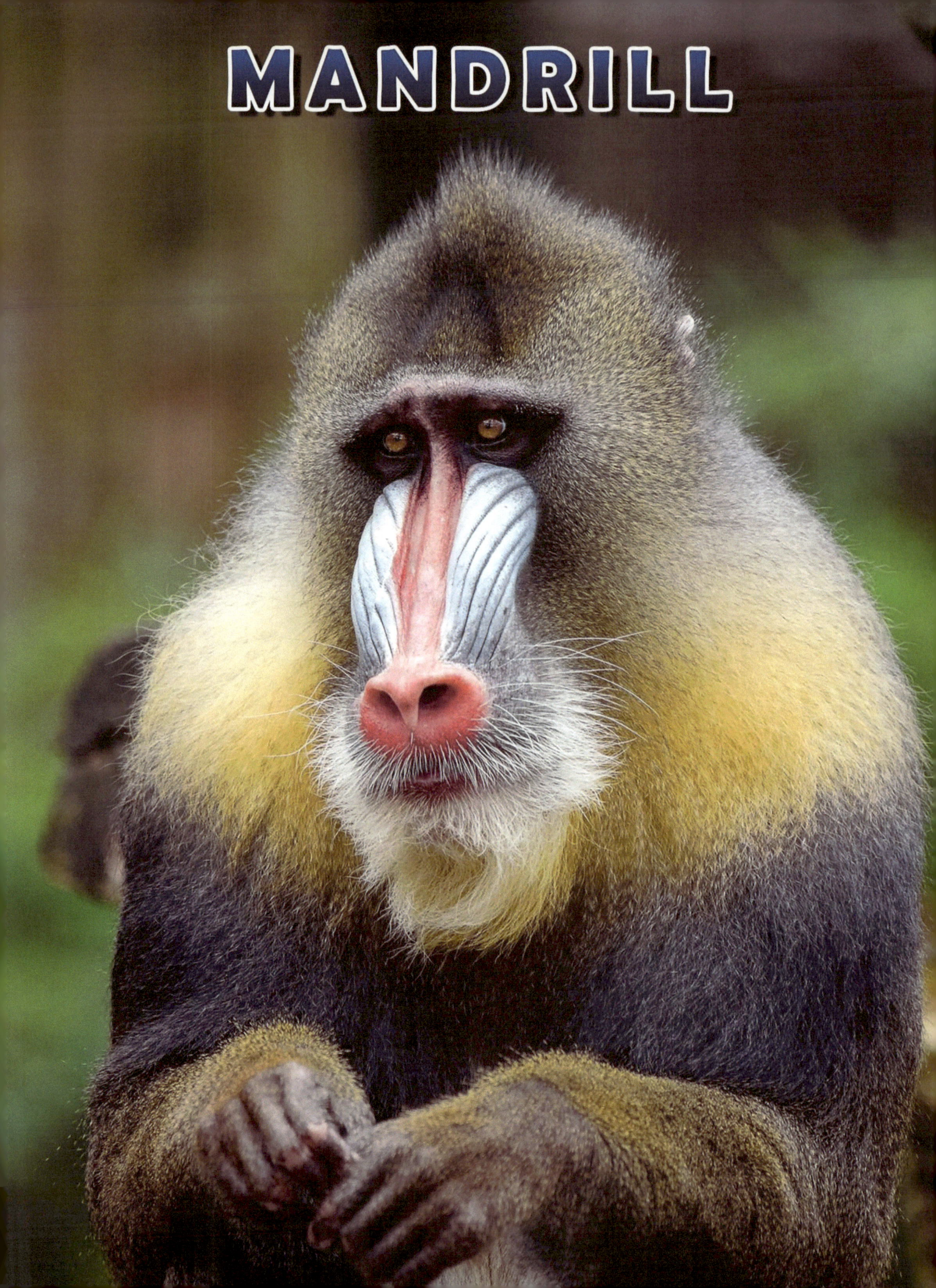

LYNX

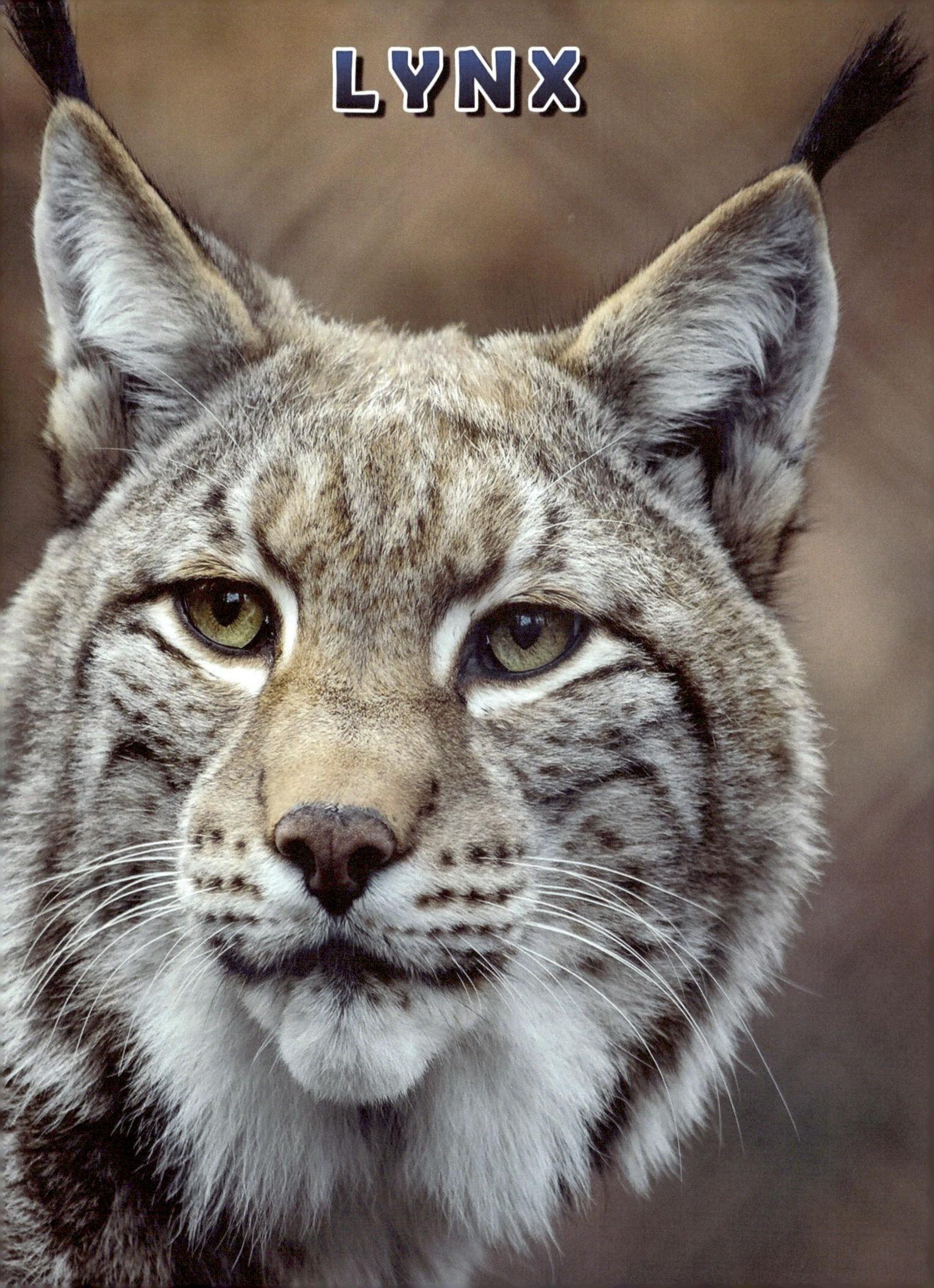

LION

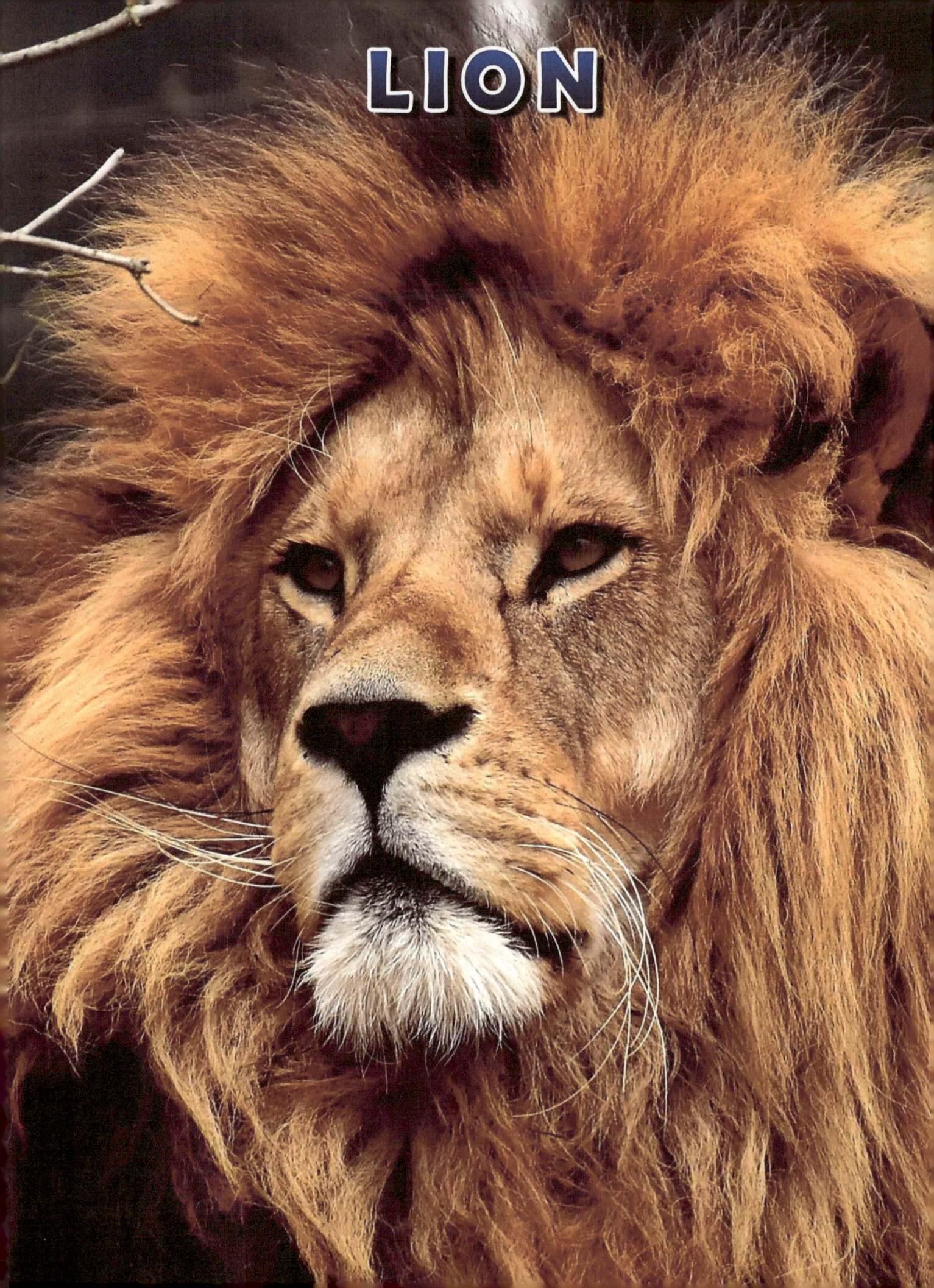

KOALAS

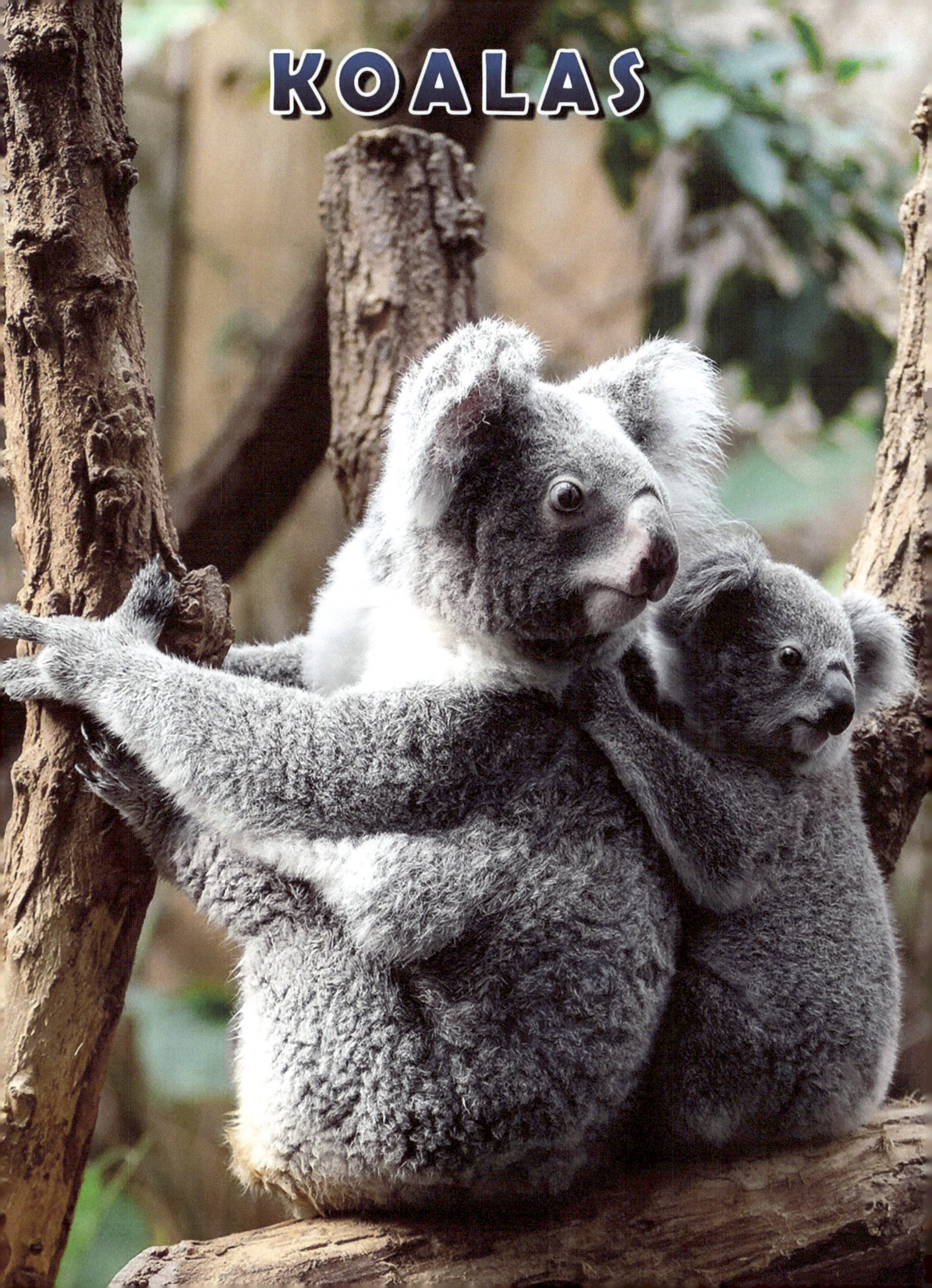

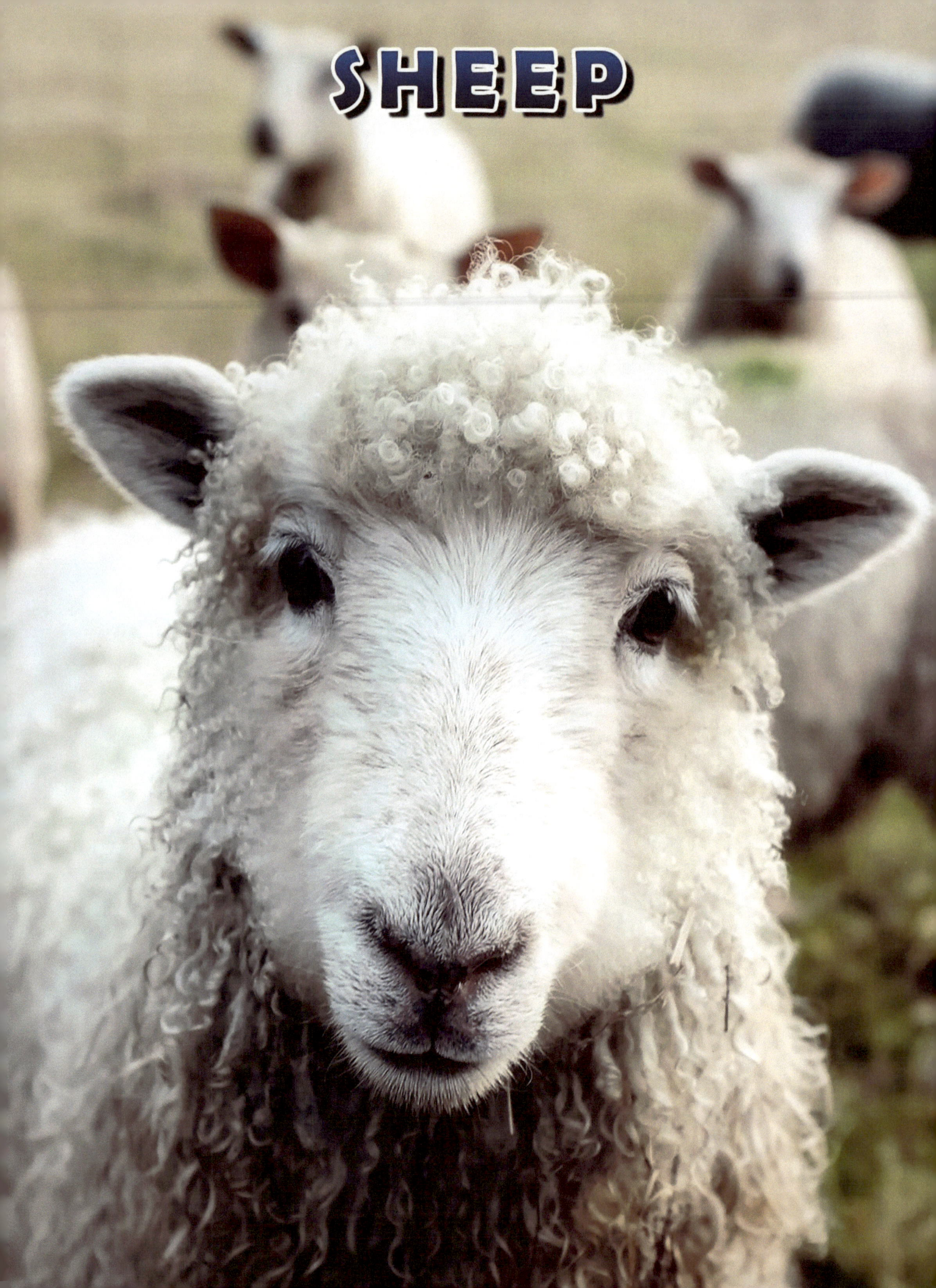

SHEEP

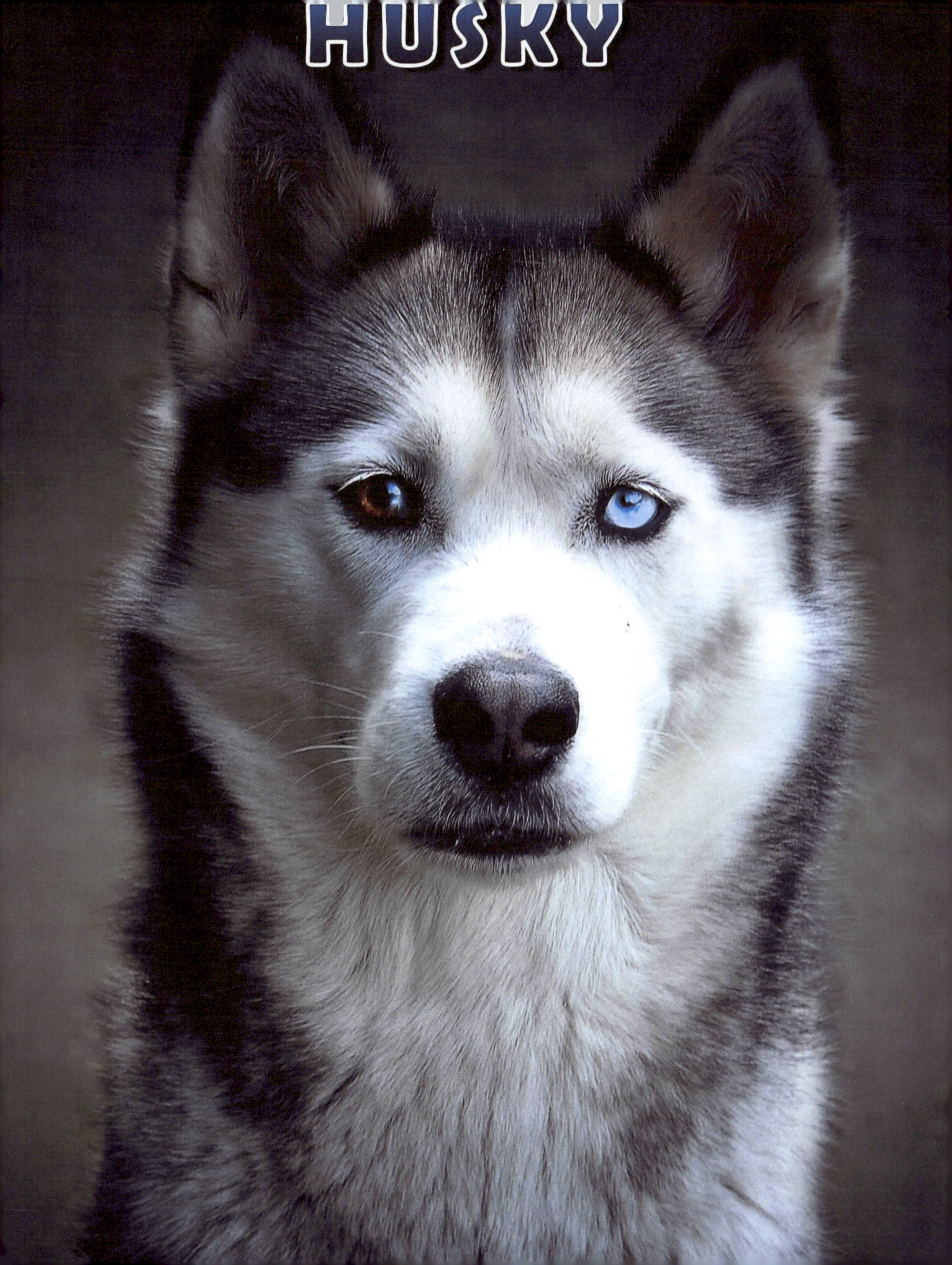

HUSKY

HUMMINGBIRD

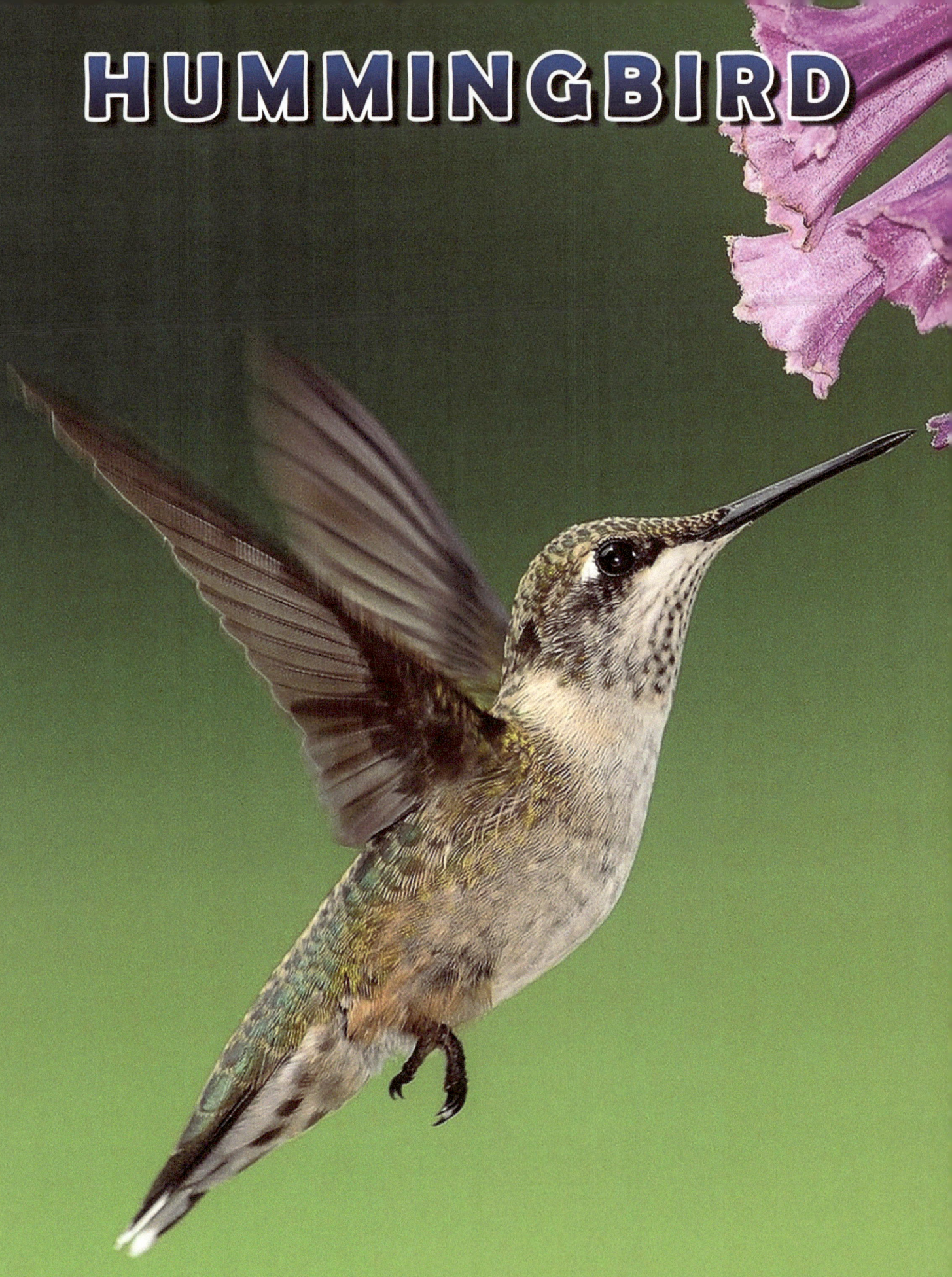

GYRFALCON

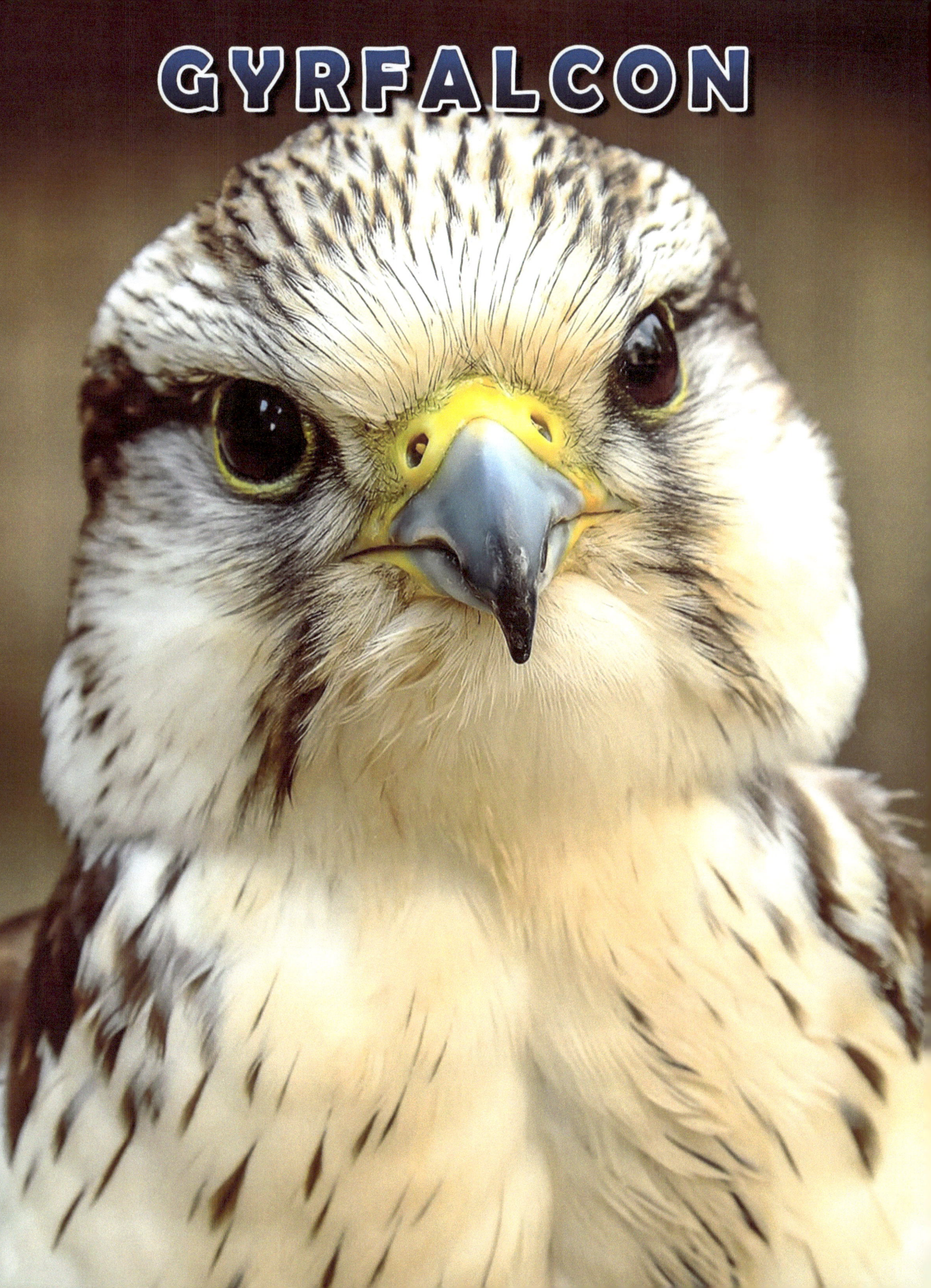

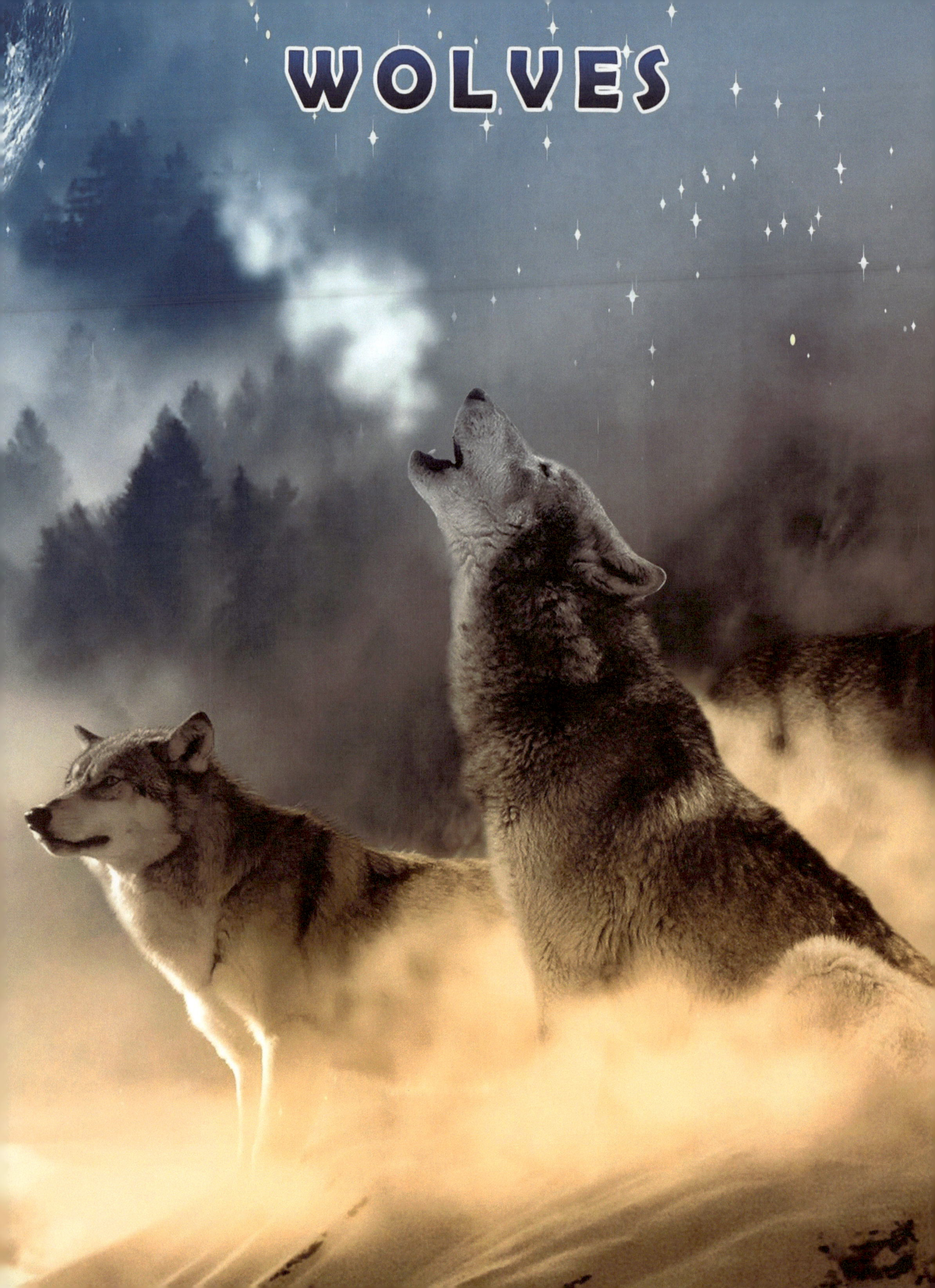

WOLVES

TIGER

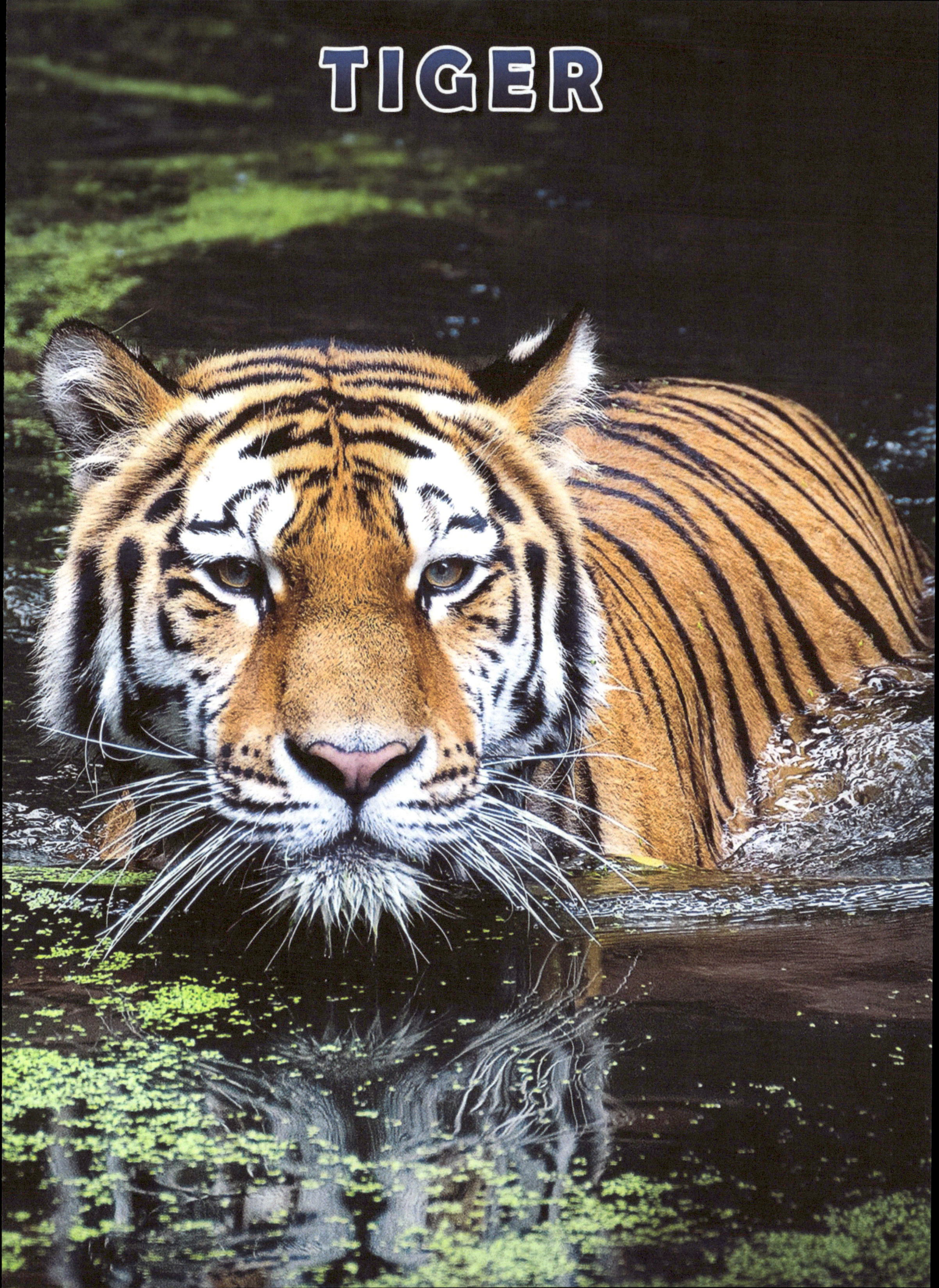

SEAGULL

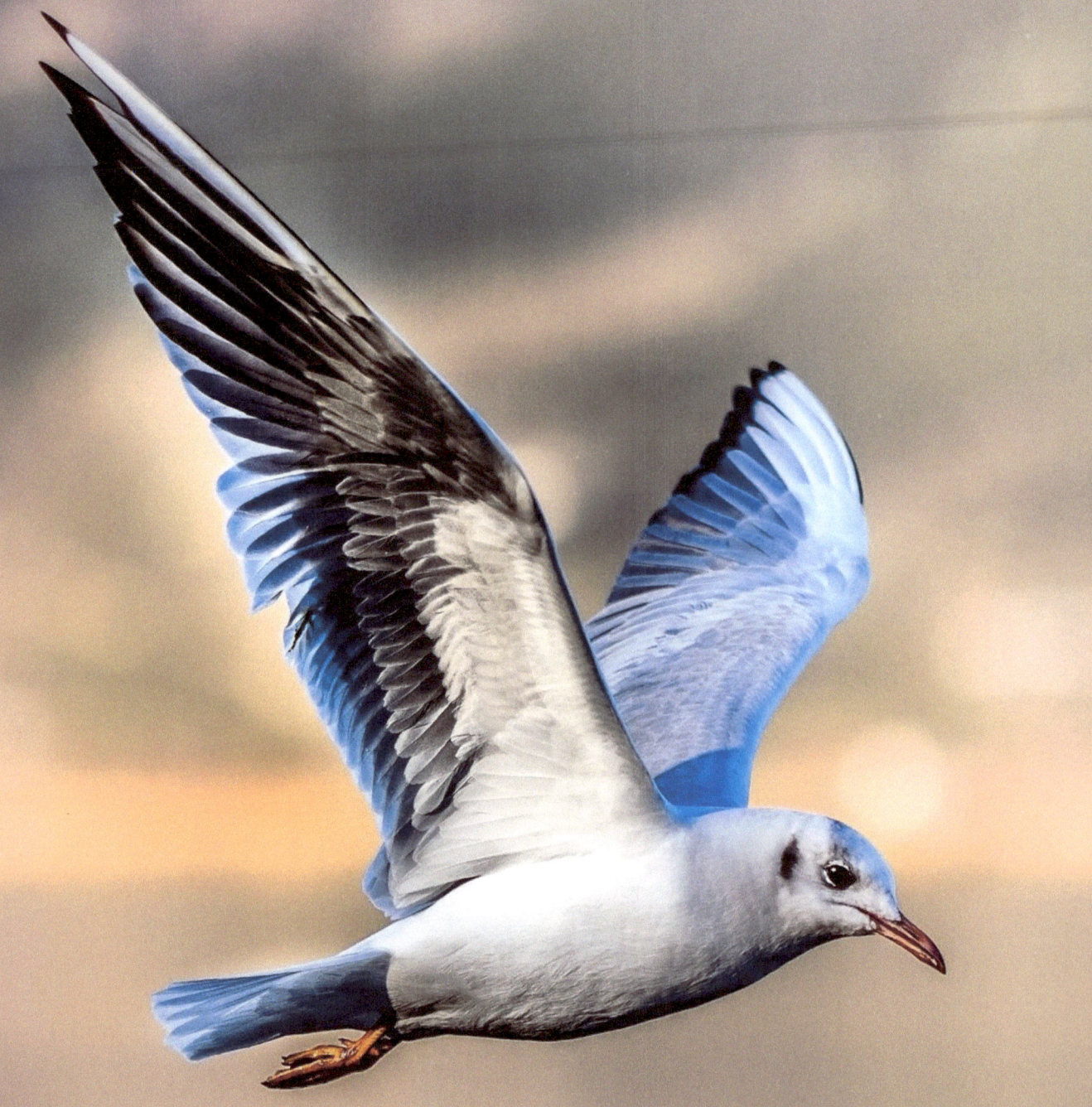

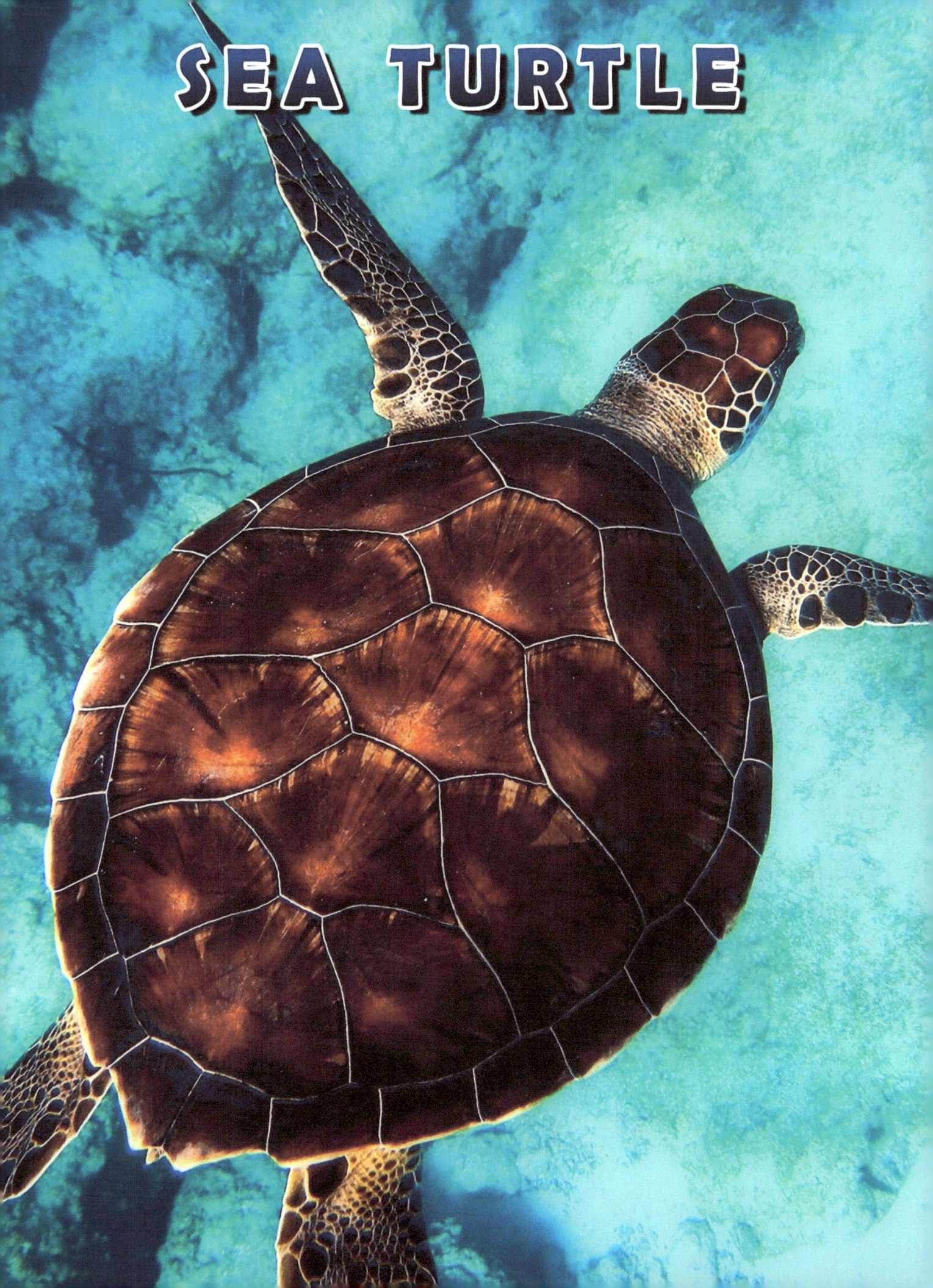

SEA TURTLE

RAINBOW LORIKEET

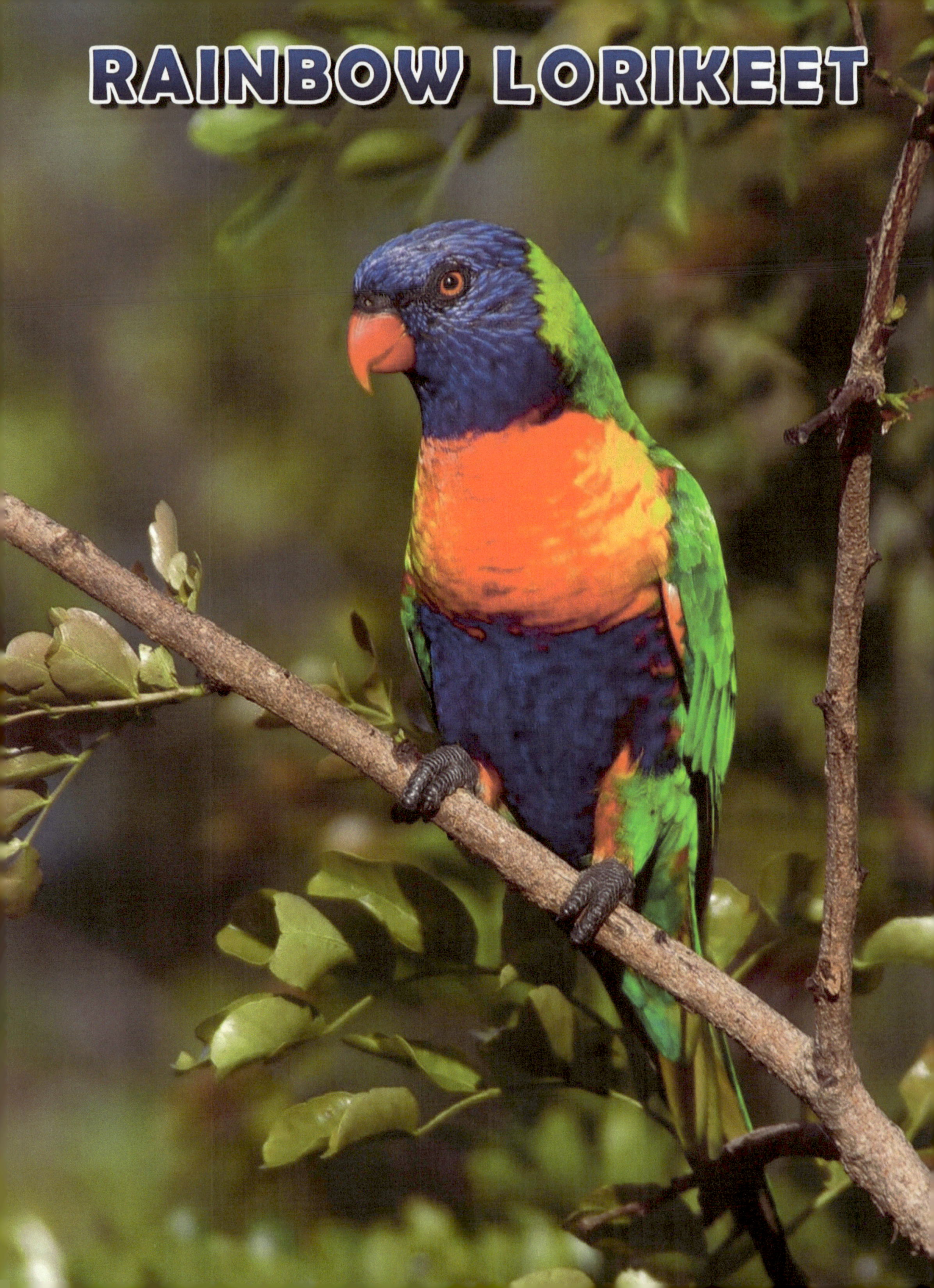

RABBIT

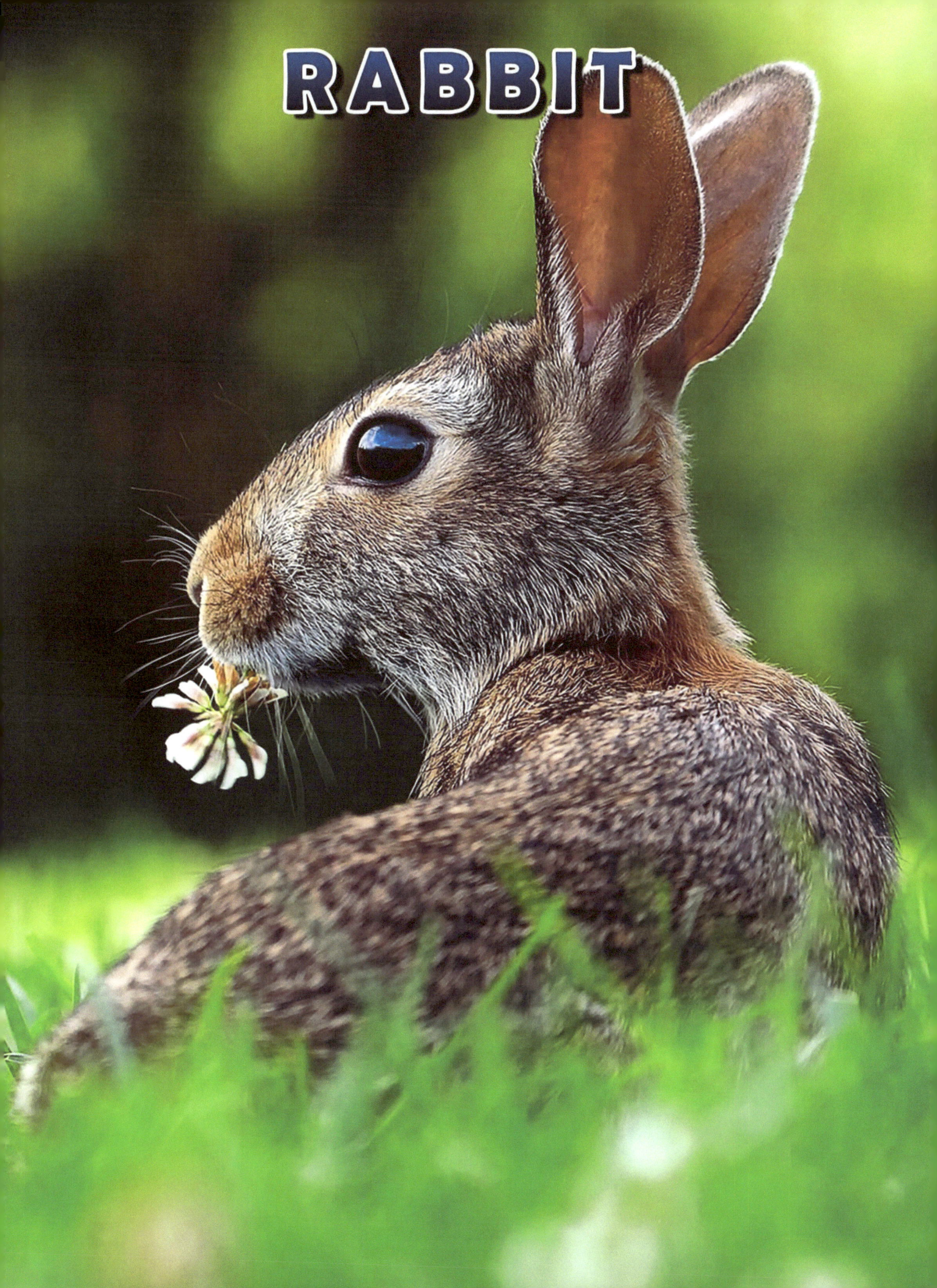

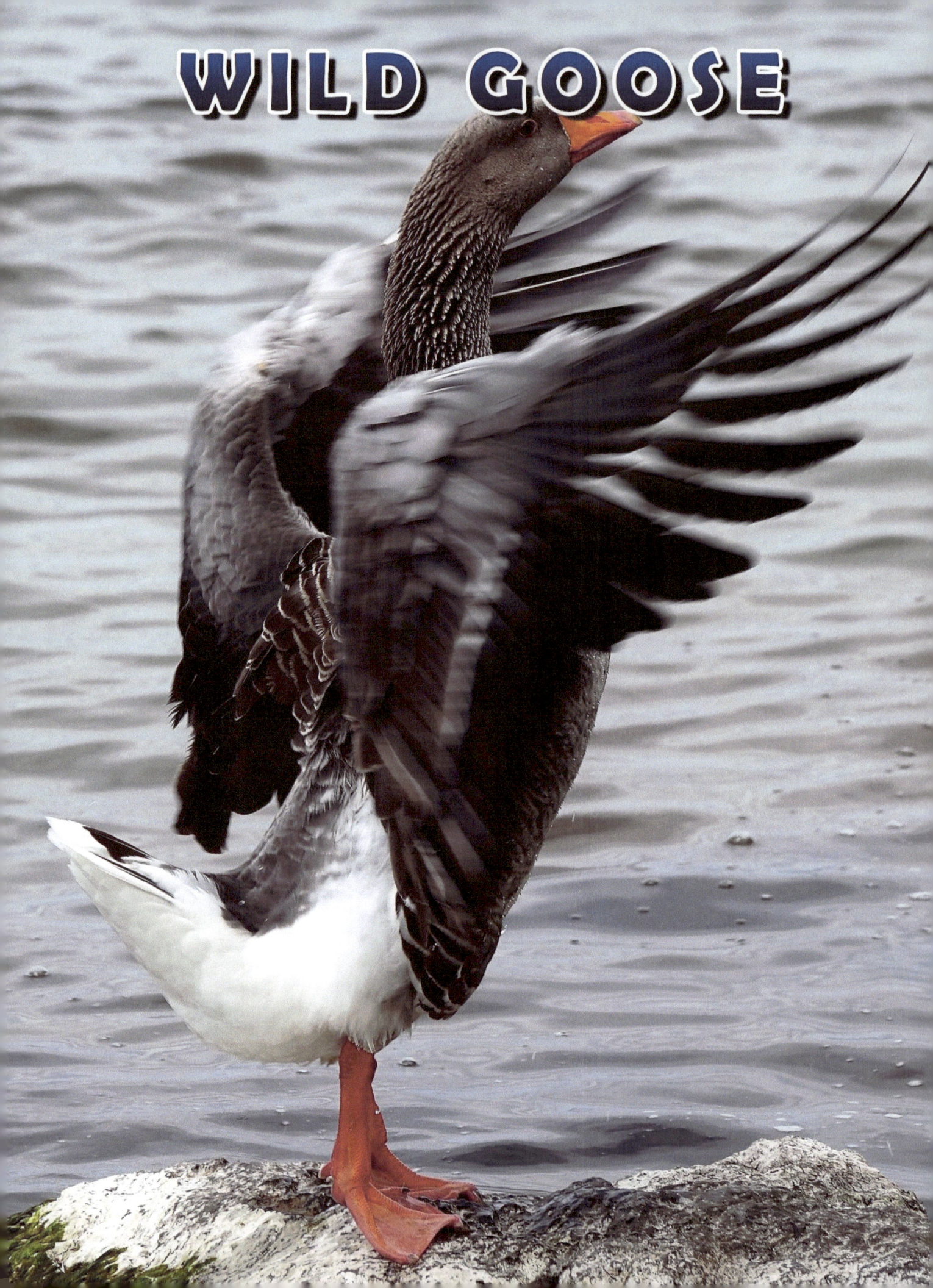

WILD GOOSE

HORSE

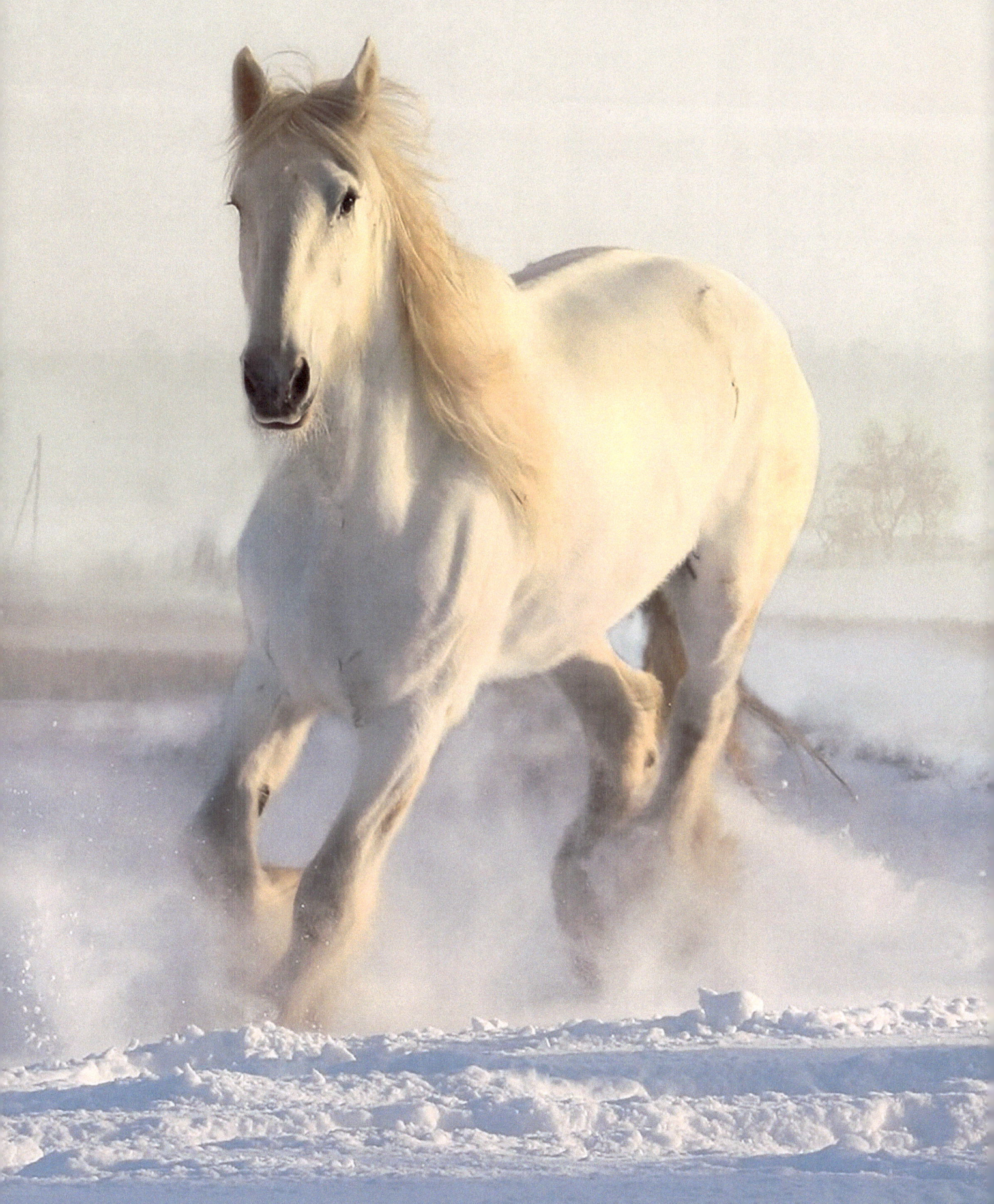

SQUIRREL

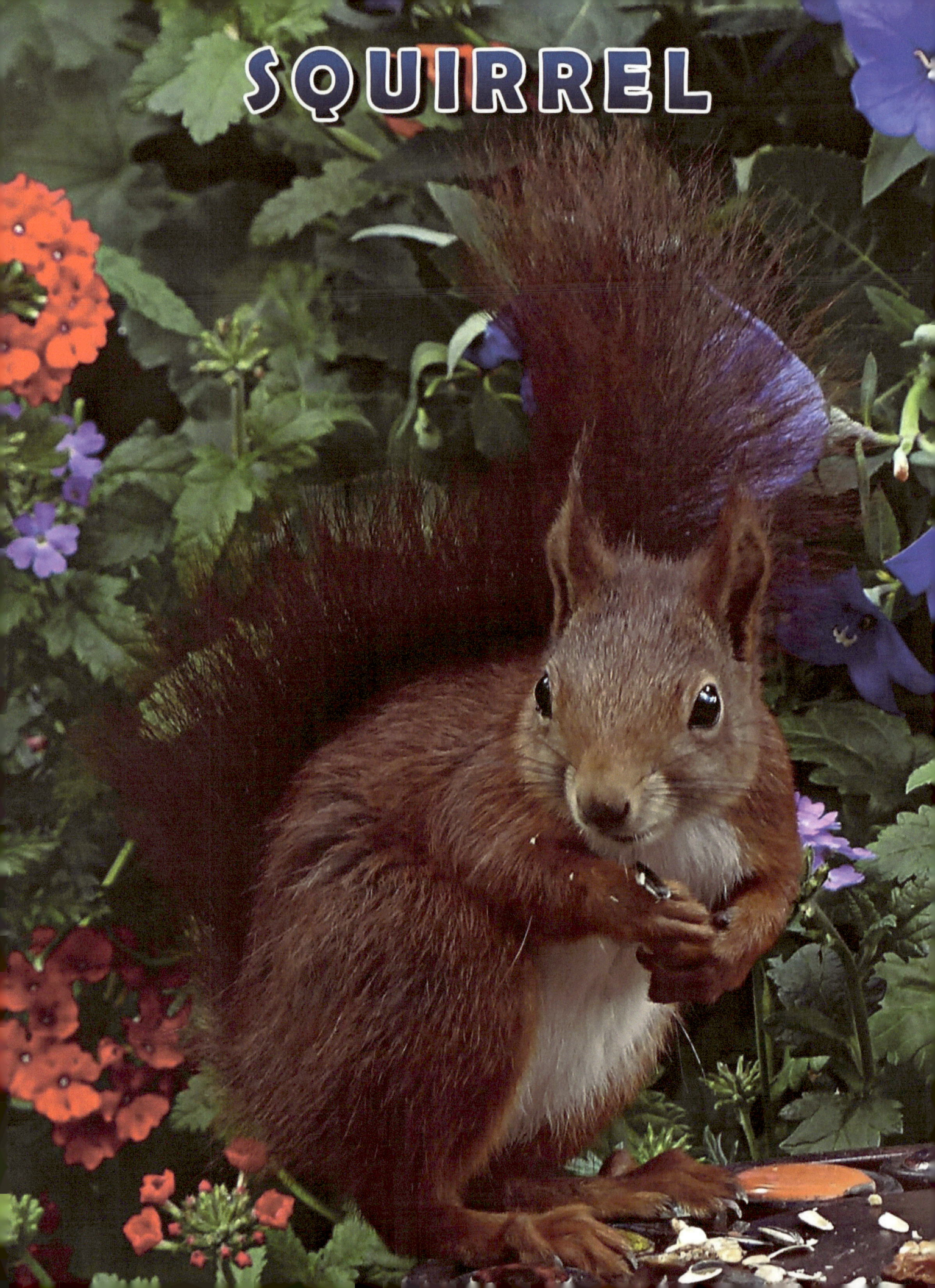

RACCOON

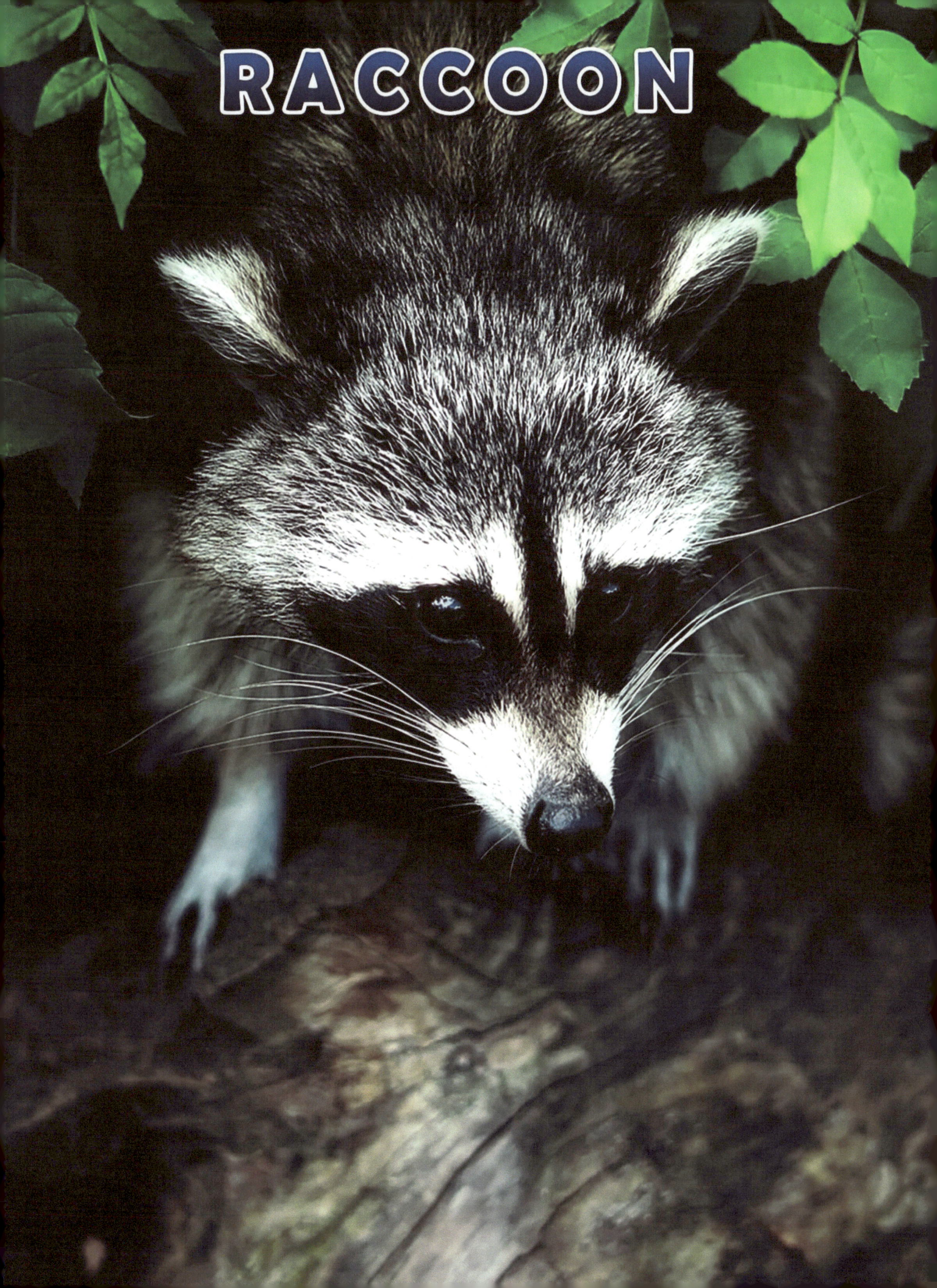

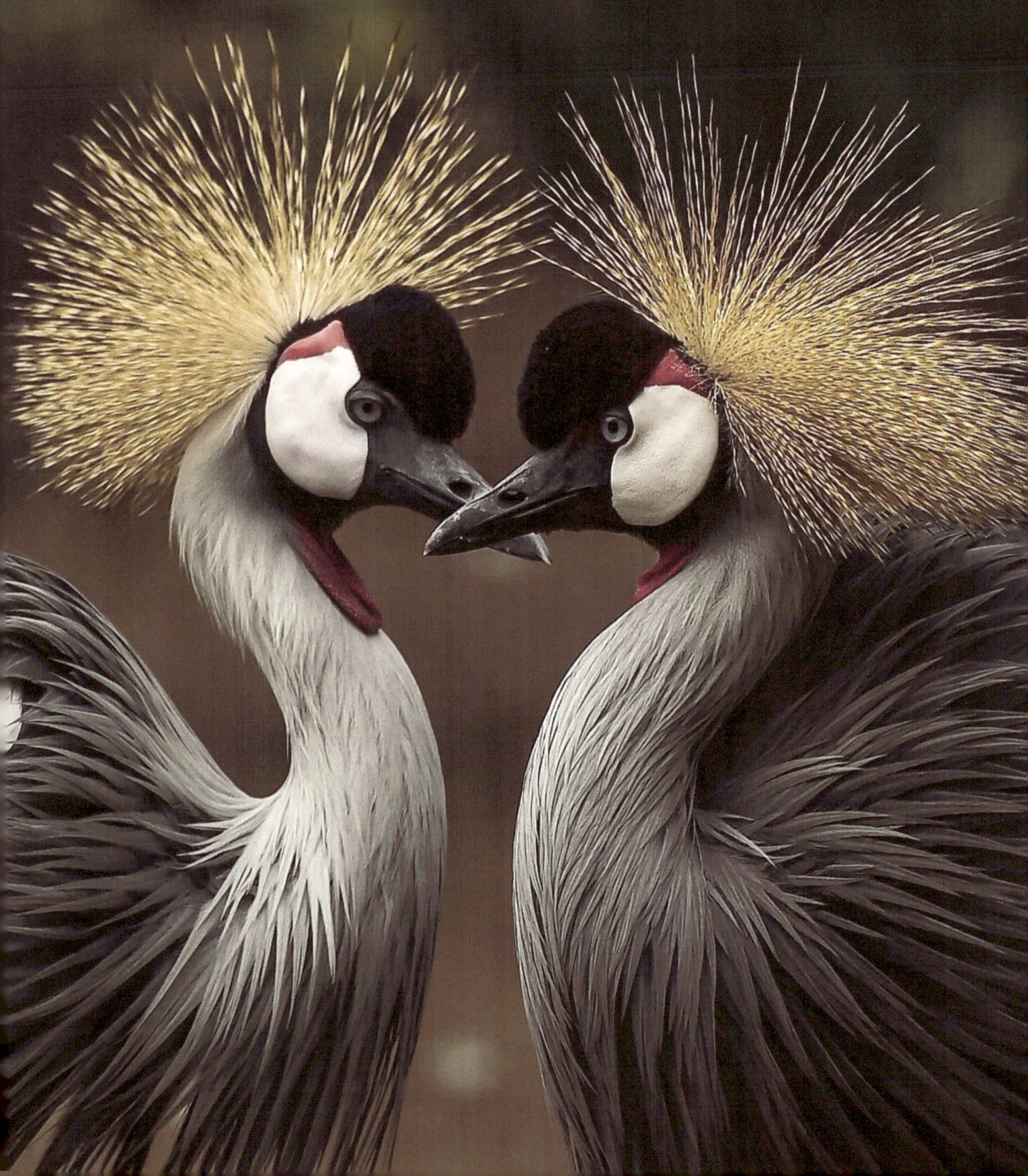

GREY CROWNED CRANES

DEER

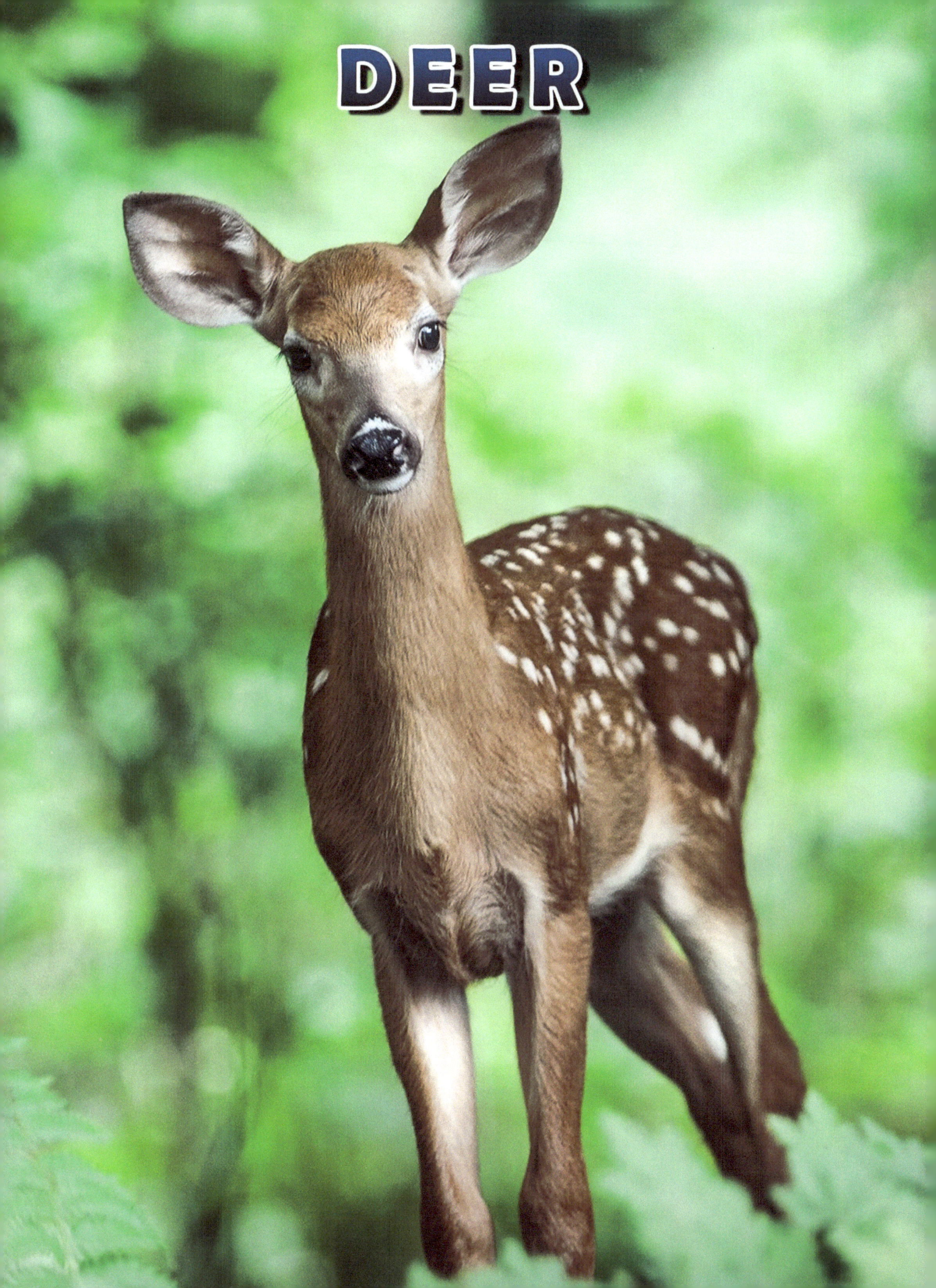

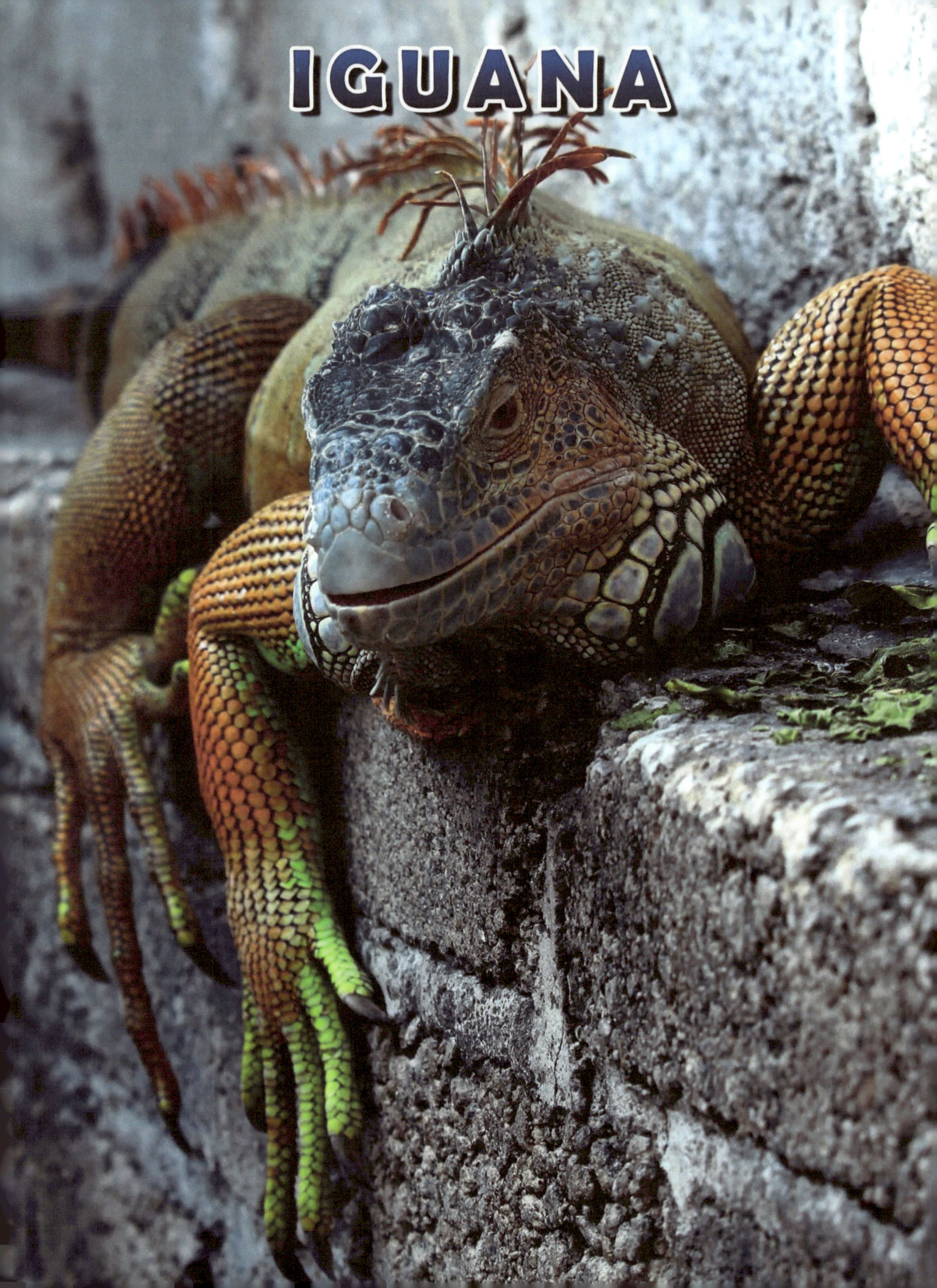

IGUANA

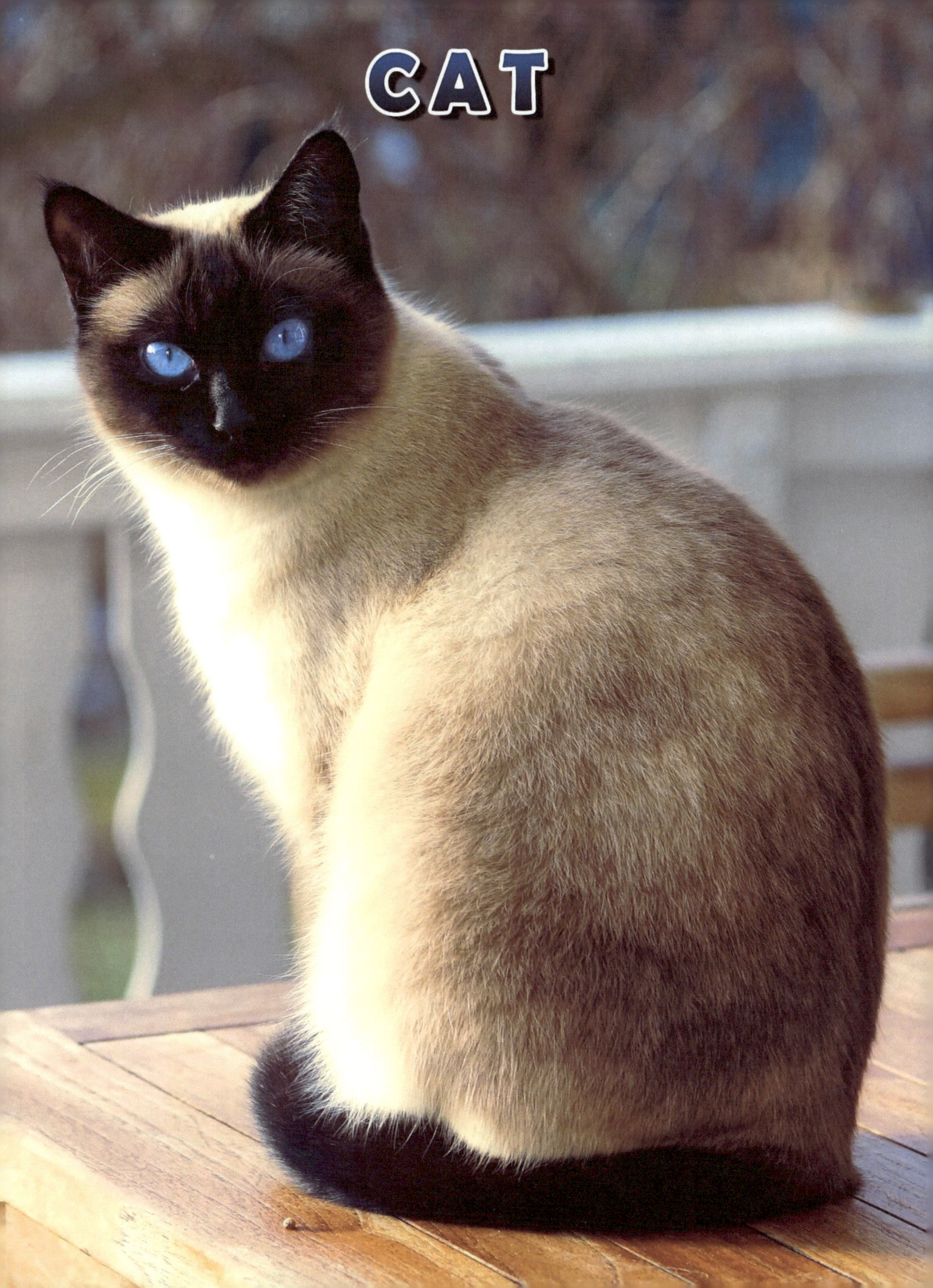

CAT

FANTASTIC

THANK YOU FOR BUYING.

If you have enjoyed this book, please tell your friends.

For more books, please visit: etidbitz.com/books

ANIMALS

www.ingramcontent.com/pod-product-compliance
Lightning Source LLC
Chambersburg PA
CBHW041523280526
45792CB00004B/1361